ESSENTIALS

OF *Gastrointestinal*

Radiology

BRONWYN JONES, F.R.A.C.P., F.R.C.R.

Assistant Professor of Radiology, The
Russell H. Morgan Department of Radiology
and Radiological Sciences, Johns Hopkins
University School of Medicine.
Radiologist, Johns Hopkins Hospital

JOHN M. BRAVER, M.D.

Radiologist, Brigham and Women's Hospital
Instructor, Harvard Medical School

1982

W. B. SAUNDERS COMPANY

PHILADELPHIA/LONDON/TORONTO/MEXICO CITY/RIO DE JANEIRO/SYDNEY/TOKYO

W. B. Saunders Company: West Washington Square
Philadelphia, PA   19105

1 St. Anne's Road
Eastbourne, East Sussex BN21 3UN, England

1 Goldthorne Avenue
Toronto, Ontario M8Z 5T9, Canada

Cedro 512
Mexico 4, D.F., Mexico

Rua Coronel Cabrita, 8
Sao Cristovao Caixa Postal 21176
Rio de Janeiro, Brazil

9 Waltham Street
Artarmon, N.S.W. 2064, Australia

Ichibancho, Central Bldg., 22-1 Ichibancho
Chiyoda-Ku, Tokyo 102, Japan

Essentials of Gastrointestinal Radiology   ISBN   0-7216-5207-7

Last digit is the print number: 9   8   7   6   5   4   3   2   1

For all the residents who have cried abjectly,
"But isn't there a small book on GI?"

PREFACE

The newcomer to gastrointestinal radiology is immediately faced with many problems requiring simultaneous solution: how to choose the proper examination for a given patient's particular problems; how to actually perform the appropriate examination, i.e., what machinery to use and how to use it; what contrast agents (if any) to select; how to obtain appropriate radiographs; and last, but by no means least, how to interpret the finished study. There is no basic comprehensive text to guide the neophyte through this complex maze; it is our intention to provide the budding radiologist with the tools necessary to perform and to successfully interpret the appropriate examination. This is not meant to be an encyclopedic treatise on gastrointestinal disease; rather it will focus on basic principles and their application. The reader can then turn to other available sources for a more in-depth discussion of a particularly interesting subject.

Although there are obvious structural and physiologic differences among various parts of the gastrointestinal tract, this portion of our anatomy is unique in that, to paraphrase an old saying, the more things are different, the more they are the same. It is useful to think of the entire tract as a hollow muscular tube made up of the same basic layers. Some pathologic processes may be more common in one or another area, but "a tube is a tube is a tube," and a wide range of disease processes not only can occur anywhere along this tract, but *each disease process* will have *similar radiographic manifestations* regardless of where it occurs.

To illustrate this generalization, let us look at ulcer formation. The pathologic process of ulcer formation includes disruption of mucosa, penetration into submucosa, and edema. The basic radiographic appearance of an ulcer will thus be identical whether that ulcer occurs in the esophagus, stomach, duodenum, small bowel, or colon. Once the basic principles are learned and the expected radiographic appearance is deduced from them, we can diagnose an ulcer wherever it occurs by applying these few salient principles.

The introductory chapter demonstrates how a working knowledge of anatomy and embryology can be useful in everyday diagnosis. The basic hardware used to produce images is briefly considered. In Chapter 2, a more detailed discussion of the approach to the routine case follows step by step, from patient preparation, selection of proper contrast agent, and performance of the examination, to final interpretation. We will attempt to answer frequently recurring questions, such as: What is the expected yield of this study? What are its limitations? In the following chapter (Chapter 3), this step-by-step approach is again used in a more difficult examination: the emergency patient.

By this time, we hope the neophyte will have a good working knowledge of the basics and we will now apply this knowledge to specific disease entities. We have chosen to forgo the usual strictly anatomic approach to diagnosis and propose to group disease entities into certain broad categories which make sense *radiographically* in view of many obvious similarities. Hence we will emphasize the similar radiographic appearances of many different neoplastic diseases and study common tumors as a group. Some diseases have undoubtedly been "squeezed" into a major category, but we believe all groupings make sense from a *radiologic* viewpoint.

This is meant to be a beginner's guidebook and relates primarily to contrast radiography performed in the GI suite. However, we recognize the increasing importance of ancillary disciplines, both radiologic (computed tomography, ultrasound, nuclear medicine, angiography) and nonradiologic (endoscopy). Our purpose in this book is not the interpretation of these studies per se, but rather a description of their role in the diagnostic workup.

In this spirit, we have constructed the biliary/pancreatic section as an exercise in the diagnostic approach to the patient with a particular problem. How should the workup of a patient with a particular set of symptoms and a suspected diagnosis proceed? The general diagnostic radiologist's role in the selection of appropriate contrast studies is stressed, as well as the indications for, and the appropriate sequence of, ancillary studies.

If you have come to the conclusion that the intact gastrointestinal tract is difficult enough to study, you may well be overwhelmed by examining the postoperative patient. A discussion of common post-surgical conditions is presented with the view in mind that if the radiologist understands what was done at surgery and how and why the anatomy was altered, then he or she will understand what is seen on the radiographs.

We have included a chapter on pseudolesions because all radiologists, and especially beginners, are frequently misled by both intrinsic and extrinsic artifacts, which can be confused with pathology.

No work of this kind can be encyclopedic, and we have deliberately chosen not to be. For more in-depth study, we have appended useful references. We believe, however, that the material we have presented will form a solid foundation in modern gastrointestinal radiology.

ACKNOWLEDGMENTS

We would like to thank our secretary, Faith Hulse, and her able associates, Judith Lopez, Nancy Harrison, and Mary Slater, for their secretarial skills and their patience and forbearance over the months, especially during the final push.

We would like to especially thank Thomas Moon of Boston, whose splendid photography greatly enhances the quality of this book.

CONTENTS

1

ANATOMY

A thorough understanding of anatomy is essential both for performing radiologic examinations and for interpreting the radiographs correctly. Obviously the subject is so vast we can only highlight some areas particularly pertinent to our everyday work. Newer cross-sectional techniques (computed tomography and ultrasound) have made anatomy in general, and organ relationships in particular, easier to understand, and these will be illustrated.

EMBRYOLOGY

The *embryology* of the gut is complicated, but some basic knowledge is helpful in deciphering anatomic structure as diverse as that seen in congenital malformations and the blood supply of particular organs. The pharynx, esophagus, stomach, and proximal duodenum all originate from the foregut; the midgut gives rise to the remainder of the duodenum, all the small bowel and the colon up to midtransverse. The remainder of the colon is of hindgut origin.

The sequence of development of the large and small bowel is particularly complex, but understanding certain salient features will make interpretation of gastrointestinal (GI) studies easier. The GI tract is originally a single tube consisting of respiratory and neural elements as well as gut epithelium. This tube subsequently differentiates by a complex series of steps; these include separation, canalization, obliteration of the lumen, and recanalization. *Failure of separation* can occur, resulting in such diverse lesions as tracheoesophageal fistula, neuroenteric cyst,

and duplication, which can vary from small cyst-like structures to a completely paired organ, such as a double colon. *Failure of recanalization* causes varying degrees of atresia, the most common of which is duodenal atresia in Down's syndrome. *Regression* of structures also occurs during development of the gut, as it does in the aortic arches. For example, pancreatic tissue originally surrounds the descending duodenum; if regression does not take place, an annular pancreas will result, which may cause duodenal obstruction.

Two other basic processes occur during the development of the GI tract: *rotation* and *fixation*. If one or both do not occur normally, the abnormality can be readily documented with contrast studies and occasionally by a plain abdominal film alone. During embryogenesis the gut herniates out of and then back into the abdominal cavity. While outside, the midgut rotates 270 degrees counterclockwise and then returns to the abdomen; thus, the root of the mesentery becomes *fixed*, with one end at the ligament of Treitz and the other in the right iliac fossa. The colon returns next: the distal large bowel first, the cecum last. The colon wraps itself around the central small bowel and becomes fixed around the edge of the abdomen, forming a "picture frame" for the small bowel.

Errors in this complex process can be grave, such as an omphalocele, or less crucial, such as a variant of malrotation; for instance, the cecum may remain in the right upper quadrant (cecal arrest). In the neonate, this can result in duodenal obstruction, when thin strands of tissue (Ladd's bands) run from this misplaced cecum across the duodenal sweep and compress it. Arrest can occur at any stage,

1

and thus the radiographic appearance can be predicted. This is not entirely a trivial matter. For example, a patient with a rotation error that results in the colon being on the left (the small bowel would be on the right) will not present with classic right lower quadrant findings if he develops appendicitis. Even more serious conditions can result from improper rotation and mesenteric fixation, such as cecal volvulus in adults or the lethal midgut volvulus of infants.

Knowledge of embryology also aids comprehension of the arterial supply to the gut. Different segments of gut should have roughly the same blood supply if they derive from the same precursor. Thus, midgut organs (small bowel to midtransverse colon) are supplied by branches of the superior mesenteric artery while the remainder of the colon (hindgut origin) is supplied by the inferior mesenteric artery. Anastomoses between the two systems are crucial in preventing ischemia of the colon when flow through either major vessel is compromised.

NORMAL ANATOMY

ESOPHAGUS. The esophagus is a muscular tube some 25 cm long; in the upper third its circular muscle is striated, in the lower two thirds it is smooth. The radiologic importance of this anatomic/physiologic fact becomes ob-

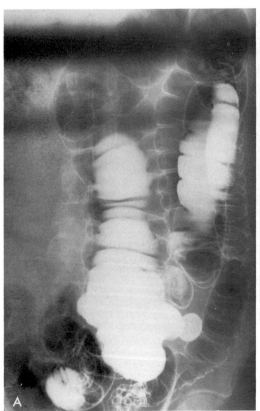
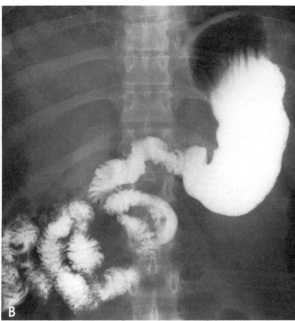

Figure 1–1. *A, Nonrotation:* Barium enema demonstrates that all the colon is situated in the left side of the abdominal cavity. The cecum is in the midabdomen and is not fixed in its normal position in the right lower quadrant. All the small bowel is in the right side of the abdomen. *B, Nonrotation of the duodenum:* A small bowel series shows that the ligament of Treitz is not in the normal position — namely, just to the left of the first lumbar vertebra. The duodenal C-sweep is not a C at all, and the proximal jejunum, instead of being in the left midabdomen, is in the right midabdomen. This finding of nonrotation of the duodenum can be an isolated one, or it can be associated with other rotational anomalies. Always check where the ligament of Treitz is, or you will miss either a rotational abnormality or a mass causing displacement.

vious on examining patients with scleroderma. This disease involves smooth muscle, so normal peristalsis would be expected in the upper third of the esophagus with absent or abnormal peristalsis in the distal two thirds; this can be verified fluoroscopically on barium swallow. Patients with diseases of striated muscle, on the other hand, such as polymyositis or myasthenia gravis, may have a combination of *pharyngeal* and *upper esophageal* motility disorders.

A thorough knowledge of the relationships of all structures impinging on the esophagus is crucial to the interpretation of normal and pathologic indentations on the barium-filled esophagus. Several examples will serve to stress this point. The cervical esophagus is closely applied to the cervical spine with only a few millimeters of thin areolar prevertebral (retropharyngeal) soft tissue between it and the vertebral bodies. Hematomas or abscesses will enlarge this prevertebral soft tissue space and push the esophagus forward; bubbles of air in these soft tissues make the diagnosis of an abscess likely (Fig. 1–2). In the thorax, the esophagus is intimately related to the trachea and the lung roots (Fig. 1–3). Spread of neoplasm or infection from one organ to another is facilitated not only because of this intimate relationship but also because the esophagus has no serosa; there is thus one less barrier to the spread of disease. Similarly, tracheoesophageal fistulas can result and inflammatory processes in carinal lymph nodes can distort the esophageal wall, resulting in the characteristic traction diverticulum.

A three-dimensional mental image of the relationship of one organ to another is critical to an understanding of how the gastrointestinal tract will be displaced by enlargement of other abdominal organs and how disease spreads within the abdominal cavity. The cross-sectional display obtained by computed tomography is especially helpful in visualizing these relationships.

For all intents and purposes, only the left lobe of the liver lies *anterior* to the stomach. Thus, if the stomach is displaced *posteriorly*, it is usually by enlargement of the left lobe of the liver; an enlarged spleen will tend to displace the stomach medially. Remember also that the gastric fundus is very close to the undersurface of the left hemidiaphragm; separation of fundus and diaphragm suggests a pathologic process in the subphrenic space, such as an abscess.

Many structures lie *posterior* to the stomach, but probably the one of most concern clinically is the pancreas (Fig. 1–4B). A large mass in the pancreas (benign or malignant) will tend to displace the stomach *anteriorly* and perhaps superiorly. A cross-table lateral film may thus be helpful in the patient suspected of having pancreatic disease.

A three-dimensional mental image of the stomach and duodenum will also help in performing upper GI contrast examinations. The

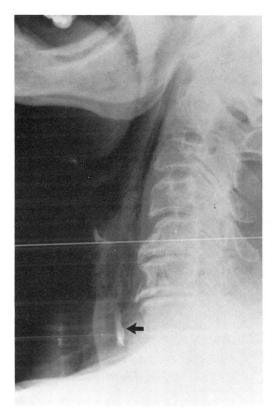

Figure 1–2. *Perforated cervical esophagus.* There is air in the retropharyngeal tissues dissecting in the prevertebral soft tissues. The chicken bone responsible for this is marked by an arrow. This calcification is too low to be part of the laryngeal cartilages. Incidentally, note the degenerative changes in the cervical spine.

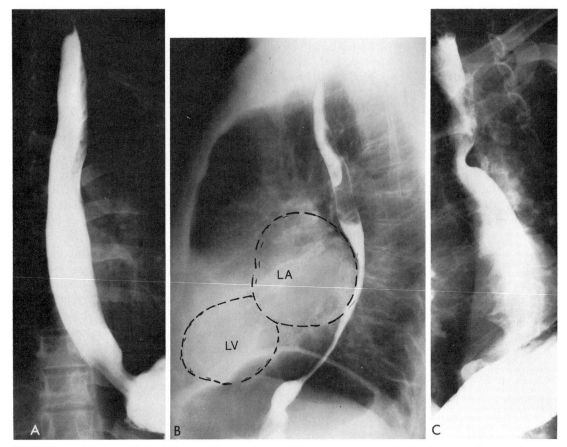

Figure 1–3. *A, Normal indentations on the esophagus.* The commonest extrinsic defect on the esophagus is from the aortic arch and this becomes more prominent with age. One can also see indentations from the left main-stem bronchus and the left atrium. *B,* When the impression from the left atrium is very obvious, as is the case here, one should suspect mitral valve disease. *C, Aberrant right subclavian artery.* There is an indentation on the posterior border of the upper third of the esophagus; this is made by an aberrant *right* subclavian artery which comes off the *left* side of the aorta; it must pass behind the esophagus to reach the right side of the neck, and thus it impinges on the esophagus.

object here is to manipulate contrast material and air into appropriate parts of a viscus; remember, barium will sink, air will rise. For example, when the patient is erect, the greater curvature of the stomach is dependent, so barium will pool there. With the patient supine, barium will pool in the gastric fundus because the fundus is posterior. Conversely, with the patient prone, the fundus will empty of barium and fill with air, and the barium will now run into the antrum. Positioning is important not only to obtain appropriate views (e.g., left side down to fill the right-sided antrum with air), but also to empty the stomach of barium. If a patient is given barium and left on his back, all the barium will stay in the fundus; he must be rolled onto his right side for the stomach to empty. If this is not done, a false diagnosis of gastric outlet obstruction may be made. Similarly, pooling of oral cholecystographic contrast material in the fundus of an immobile patient is a common cause of "nonvisualization" of the gallbladder.

PATHWAYS OF SPREAD OF DISEASE

The stomach is supported by ligaments, which are of more than casual interest. As Meyers has shown, these ligaments are one pathway for the spread of metastatic disease

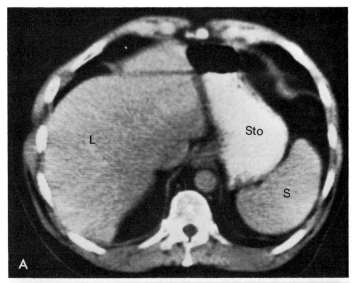

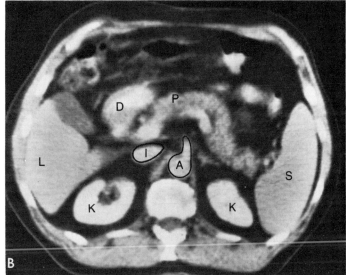

Figure 1–4. *A, Computed tomogram through the liver.* The liver (*L*) occupies the right upper abdomen; note its relationship to the contrast-filled stomach (*Sto*). The spleen (*S*) occupies a similar position in the left upper quadrant. *B, Computed tomogram through the pancreas.* This view is taken at the level of the inferior margins of the liver (*L*) and spleen (*S*) and the middle of the kidneys (*K*). The pancreas (*P*) is clearly defined in the mid-abdomen with the splenic vessels running along its posterior surface. The aorta (*A*) and inferior vena cava (*I*) are outlined, as is the origin of the superior mesenteric artery from the aorta. There is contrast medium in the stomach and the duodenal C-sweep (*D*); note the close relationship of the C-sweep to the head of the pancreas.

(Fig. 1–5). How and where these ligaments attach is constant and therefore serves as a means of predicting where disease will spread; which surface of an organ is involved can be a clue as to where a malignant process originated. The transverse colon is an example: cancer of the greater curvature of the stomach will spread along the gastrocolic ligament to the *superior* surface of the transverse colon, whereas a pancreatic process (either neoplastic or inflammatory) will spread along the transverse mesocolon to the *inferior* surface of the transverse colon. Occasionally a large pancreatic pseudocyst can rupture through the lesser sac into the gastrocolic ligament, result-

ing in separation of the stomach and transverse colon; these should lie parallel to each other when the patient is supine.

Similarly, the attachments of the small bowel mesentery and the peritoneal reflections explain the preferred areas of spread of both metastatic (drop metastases) and inflammatory disease within the peritoneal cavity. Common sites of involvement are (1) the right iliac fossa (along the root of the mesentery); (2) the pouch of Douglas (Blumer's shelf) (Fig. 1–6); (3) the superior surface of the sigmoid; and (4) the right paracolic gutter (the right gutter is open to the general peritoneal cavity; the left is closed).

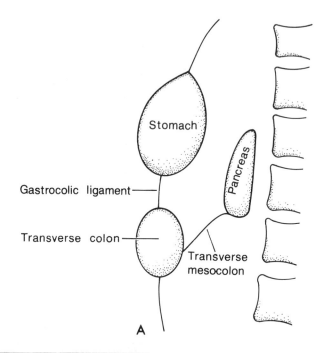

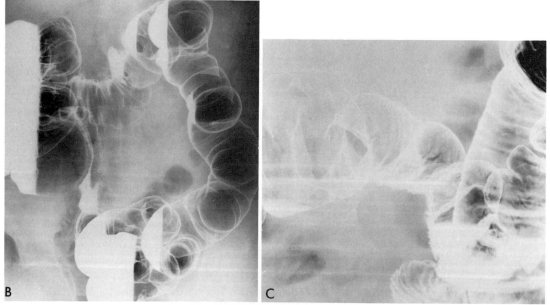

Figure 1–5. *A,* Disease may spread from organ to organ along ligaments, as described in the text. *B,* *Spread of gastric carcinoma to transverse colon.* There is spiculation and rigidity of the *superior* surface of the transverse colon due to spread of carcinoma along the gastrocolic ligament. Compare this appearance with that in *C,* in which the *inferior* surface of the transverse colon is involved by a similar process from spread of carcinoma of the pancreas.

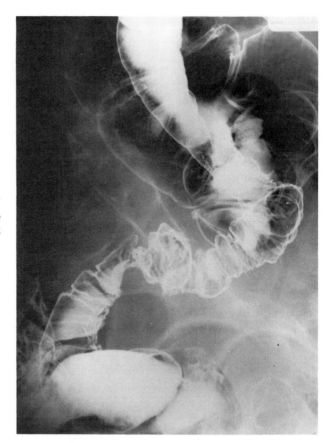

Figure 1–6. *Serosal metastases to pouch of Douglas.* There is serosal involvement of the anterior wall of the rectum, with rigidity, lack of distensibility, and spiculation.

NORMAL RADIOGRAPHIC FINDINGS

DUODENUM. Some other anatomic considerations are relevant to radiologic practice. The duodenum is divided into four parts, the first of which, the duodenal bulb, is roughly triangular in shape, faces backwards, and is intraperitoneal. The gallbladder is intimately related to the duodenal bulb, and a distended gallbladder will frequently indent the superolateral aspect of the duodenal bulb (Fig. 1–7). The close approximation of duodenal bulb and descending duodenum to the gallbladder explains the ease with which gallstones can erode into the duodenum, leading to gallstone ileus. Similarly, duodenal disease, such as an ulcer, can perforate into the biliary system via the gallbladder.

The second portion (descending) runs posteriorly parallel to the spine and is retroperitoneal, as are the third and fourth portions. The descending duodenum is also closely related to the two curvatures of the hepatic flexure; thus, carcinoma of the hepatic flexure can easily invade the descending duodenum.

The second and third portions of the duodenum constitute the "C-sweep" because they assume a configuration like the letter C. Enlargement of the head of the pancreas will cause mass effect upon the C-sweep, usually enlarging its radius of curvature (Fig. 1–8) and possibly compressing the lumen from the medial side. The right kidney is also intimately related to the descending duodenum, but a renal mass (cyst or tumor) will involve the *lateral* (outside) portion of the C-sweep.

The third (horizontal) portion of the duodenum crosses over the spine and the aorta; the superior mesenteric artery crosses over this part of the duodenum to reach the mesentery. The duodenum can become pinched between the aorta and the superior mesenteric

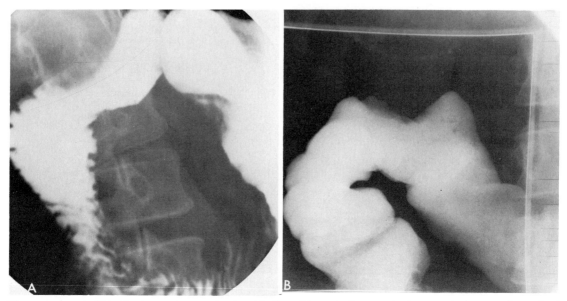

Figure 1–7. *Gallbladder impression on duodenal bulb and hepatic flexure.* A characteristic smooth extrinsic pressure defect due to the gallbladder is seen on the duodenal bulb (*A*) and hepatic flexure (*B*).

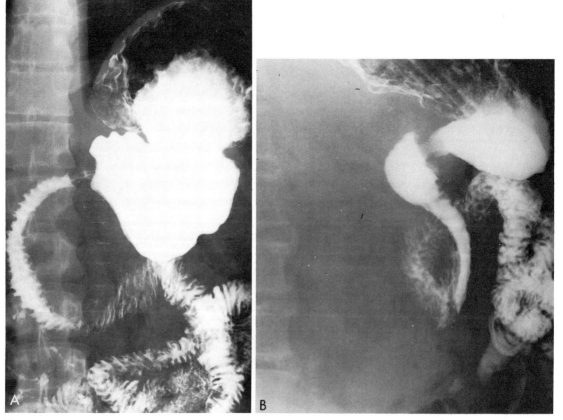

Figure 1–8. *A, Pancreatitis widening the C-sweep:* The C-sweep is enlarged from its usual tight curve, and the folds are markedly thickened but intact. *B, Displacement of the duodenum by polycystic kidneys.* On this lateral film, note the bowing and marked anterior displacement of the descending limb of the duodenum. In the normal patient, the descending limb runs parallel to and just anterior to the lumbar spine.

artery in certain individuals, resulting in duodenal obstruction — the so-called "superior mesenteric artery syndrome" (Fig. 1–9).

The fourth (ascending) portion of the duodenum climbs to the ligament of Treitz (usually to the left of the first lumbar vertebra), where the duodenum becomes the jejunum. Masses in this region (which might originate in the tail of the pancreas or the left kidney) will displace the ligament of Treitz inferiorly and usually anteriorly.

The *retroperitoneal location* of the second, third, and fourth parts of the duodenum is important to remember. With major (usually blunt) abdominal trauma, this retroperitoneal segment, because it is fixed and pressed against the spine, is prone to hemorrhage or rupture. The perforation will usually be retroperitoneal; *free* intraperitoneal air will not be visible on plain films but *retroperitoneal* air may be. The radiologist will be able to suggest this catastrophic event if the abdominal plain film is interpreted correctly.

Jejunum and Ileum. The small bowel proper, consisting of jejunum and ileum, is attached to the posterior abdominal wall by a mesentery, the root of which extends obliquely from left upper quadrant (the ligament of Treitz) to the right lower quadrant. From this relatively short attachment, the mesentery extends outwards in a series of folds to accommodate the entire length of small bowel. As has been mentioned, disease can spread along the mesentery and, if it does, this pathway can be predicted once the mesenteric anatomy is understood. In addition, it is important to point out that there are two borders to any small bowel loop: a mesenteric (fixed) and an antimesenteric (free) border (Fig. 1–10). The border facing the root of the mesentery is called *mesenteric*, whereas the border facing away from the root is called *antimesenteric*. This has certain implications, because certain diseases tend to involve one or the other border exclusively; this will be elaborated in the chapter on the small bowel.

Colon. Distinguished from the small bowel by its peripheral location and by having

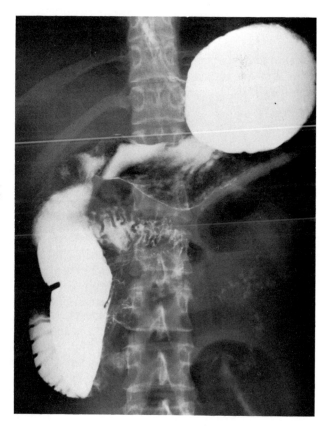

Figure 1–9. *Superior mesenteric artery syndrome:* There is marked dilatation of the proximal duodenum with a sharp linear cutoff in the horizontal limb; this is due to extrinsic compression of the duodenum by the superior mesenteric artery. Characteristically, putting the patient prone will relieve the obstruction, the prone position allowing the superior mesenteric artery to fall away from the duodenum.

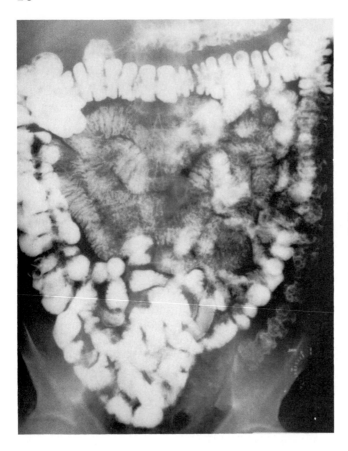

Figure 1–10. Normal small bowel and colon.

haustral folds instead of valvulae conniventes, the colon has several radiologically identifiable segments: Cecum, ascending colon, hepatic and splenic flexures, transverse, descending, and sigmoid colon, and the rectum.

The cecum is usually firmly attached in the right lower quadrant, but it (and part of the ascending colon) may have a mesentery in certain individuals and consequently be freely mobile. The ascending and descending regions of the colon are usually retroperitoneal. The transverse colon is attached by a mesentery, the transverse mesocolon, and it can be surprisingly mobile in some individuals; on barium enema it can often be seen dipping deep into the pelvis, making adequate study of this area difficult. The sigmoid colon is also attached by a mesentery of variable length; a very long mesentery predisposes to *volvulus* when the unusually mobile sigmoid twists on its axis and becomes acutely obstructed. A similar problem can occur in the cecum if the

cecum is unduly mobile because of a generous mesenteric attachment. Volvulus, a "closed loop" type of obstruction, is frequently catastrophic because of supervening vascular compromise and bowel ischemia. The radiologist can make a valuable contribution not only in diagnosis but occasionally in therapy as well; sigmoid volvulus can sometimes be reduced during a barium enema.

As in the upper GI tract, an understanding of anatomy in three dimensions is essential for performing and interpreting the barium enema. For example, the rectum and flexures are posterior, while the transverse colon is anterior. To manipulate air into the rectum, for instance, the patient should be placed prone; this simple observation frequently helps to exclude the diagnosis of complete distal colonic obstruction on plain films. Conversely, it may help to turn the patient supine to manipulate barium "over the hump" of one or both flexures. Incidentally, radiologists use the terms splenic and hepatic

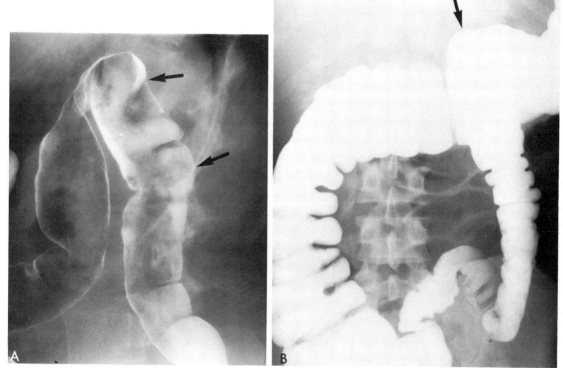

Figure 1–11. *A, Normal splenic flexure.* Note how there are in fact two flexures. The upper arrow is the radiographic flexure; the lower arrow is the anatomic flexure, where the phrenicocolic ligament is attached. *B, Renal agenesis with displacement of splenic flexure into renal bed.* A barium enema shows that the anatomic splenic flexure (arrow) is now situated medial to the radiographic splenic flexure. This occurs with left renal agenesis; it may also follow removal of the left kidney through a posterior approach if the phrenicocolic ligament is divided surgically. A similar finding can occur at the hepatic flexure in *right* renal agenesis.

flexure somewhat loosely. The *radiographic* splenic flexure is simply taken as the highest point of the colon in the left upper quadrant; the true *anatomic* splenic flexure, where the phrenicocolic ligament attaches, lies considerably more distally. Similarly, the "hepatic flexure" is actually two flexures, an anterior and a posterior one (Fig. 1–11). As we have already said, diseases involving the duodenum or masses arising in the right kidney can affect this region of the colon because of the close anatomic relationship of all these structures. Masses arising in the lower pole of the left kidney, on the other hand, characteristically do not affect the anatomic splenic flexure but do displace the descending colon laterally and anteriorly. A final point of interest is the position of the descending colon when there is congenital absence of the left kidney. In such cases, the distal transverse colon and anatomic splenic flexure lie more medial and posterior than usual, occupying the "empty" renal fossa.

References

General

Meschan I: An Atlas of Anatomy Basic to Radiology. Philadelphia, WB Saunders, 1975.

Meyers MA: Dynamic Radiology of the Abdomen: Normal and Pathological Anatomy. New York, Springer-Verlag, 1976.

Normal Anatomy

Churchill RJ, Reynes CJ, Love L, Moncada R: CT imaging of the abdomen: methodology and normal anatomy. Radiol Clin North Am 17:13–24, 1979.

Sample WF: Normal abdominal anatomy defined by gray scale ultrasound. Radiol Clin North Am 17:3–12, 1979.

Displacements and Relationships

Ghahremani GG, Meyers MA: The cholecysto-colic relationships. A roentgen-anatomic study of the colonic manifestations of gallbladder disorders. Am J Roentgenol 125:21–34, 1975.

Meyers MA: The reno-alimentary relationships. Anatomic-roentgen study of their clinical significance. Am J Roentgenol 123:386–400, 1975.

Meyers MA: Clinical involvement of mesenteric and antimesenteric borders of small bowel loops. I. Normal pattern and relationships. Gastrointest Radiol 1:41–48, 1976.

Meyers MA: Clinical involvement of mesenteric and antimesenteric borders of small bowel loops. II. Radiologic interpretation of pathologic alterations. Gastrointest Radiol 1:49–58, 1976.

Meyers MA, Whalen JP: Roentgen significance of the duodenocolic relationships: An anatomic approach. Am J Roentgenol 117:263–274, 1973.

Meyers MA, Volberg F, Katzen B, Abbott G: Haustral anatomy and pathology: A new look I. Roentgen identification of normal patterns and relationships. Radiology 108:497–504, 1973.

Meyers MA, Volberg F, Katzen B, Abbott G: Haustral anatomy and pathology: A new look. II. Roentgen interpretation of pathological alterations. Radiology 108:505–512, 1973.

Poppel MH: Duodenocolic apposition. Am J Roentgenol 83:851–856, 1960.

Whalen JP: Anatomy of the colon: guide to intra-abdominal pathology. Hickey Lecture, 1975. Am J Roentgenol 125:3–20, 1975.

Whalen JP, Evans JA, Meyers MA: Vector principle in the differential diagnosis of abdominal masses. II. Right upper quadrant. Am J Roentgenol 115:318, 1972.

Whalen JP, Evans JA, Shanser J: Vector principle in the differential diagnosis of abdominal masses. I. Left upper quadrant. Am J Roentgenol 113:104–115, 1971.

Whalen JP, Bader LM, Wolfman R: Evaluation of the retrogastric space. Normal appearance and variation. Am J Roentgenol 121:348–356, 1974.

Pathways of Spread of Disease

Meyers MA: The spread and localization of acute intraperitoneal effusions. Radiology 95:547–554, 1970.

Meyers MA: Acute extraperitoneal infection. Semin Roentgenol 8:445–453, 1973.

Meyers MA: Distribution of intra-abdominal malignant seeding: dependency on dynamics of flow of ascitic fluid. Am J Roentgenol 120:198–206, 1973.

Meyers MA, Goodman KJ: Pathways of extrapelvic spread of disease: Anatomic-radiologic correlation. Am J Roentgenol 125:900–909, 1975.

Meyers MA, Whalen JP, Peelle K, Berne AS: Radiologic features of extraperitoneal effusions. An anatomic approach. Radiology 104:249–257, 1972.

Superior Mesenteric Artery Syndrome

Gondos B: Duodenal compression defect and the "superior mesenteric artery syndrome." Radiology 123:575–580, 1977.

Malrotation

Balthazar EJ: Congenital positional anomalies of the colon: radiographic diagnosis and clinical implications. I. Abnormalities of rotation. Gastrointest Radiol 2:41–47, 1977.

Balthazar EJ: Congenital positional anomalies of the colon: radiographic diagnosis and clinical implications. II. Abnormalities of fixation. Gastrointest Radiology 2:49–56, 1977.

Firor HV, Harris VJ: Rotational abnormalities of the gut: re-emphasis of a neglected facet, isolated incomplete rotation of the duodenum. Am J Roentgenol 120:315–321, 1974.

Internal Hernias

Ghahremani GG, Meyers MA: Internal abdominal hernias. Curr Probl Radiol 5:3–30, 1975.

Meyers MA: Paraduodenal hernias. Radiologic and arteriographic diagnosis. Radiology 95:29–37, 1970.

Renal Agenesis

Curtis JA, Sadhu V, Steiner RM: Malposition of the colon in right renal agenesis, ectopia, and anterior nephrectomy. Am J Roentgenol 129:845–850, 1977.

Mascatello V, Lebowitz RL: Malposition of the colon in left renal agenesis and ectopia. Radiology 120:371–376, 1976.

Meyers MA: Roentgen significance of the phrenicocolic ligament. Radiology 95:539–545, 1970.

Meyers MA, Whalen JP, Evans JA, Viamonte M: Malposition and displacement of the bowel in renal agenesis and ectopia: new observations. Am J Roentgenol 117:323–333, 1973.

Whalen JP, Riemenschneider PA: An analysis of the normal anatomic relationships of the colon as applied to roentgenographic observations. Am J Roentgenol 99:55–61, 1967.

2

TECHNICAL ASPECTS

RADIATION TECHNOLOGY

The technology of machines and the physics of radiology tend to intimidate many physicians. Some prefer to consider the whole process a "black box" and deal only with the final product, an image on film. There are disadvantages to both patient and doctor from this ostrich-like approach, and some basic knowledge of how a film is produced for interpretation is essential for quality radiography.

The physics of x-ray production we will leave to excellent basic physics texts, and we will concentrate here on some of the hardware used to produce images in gastrointestinal radiography. The basic machinery will consist of a three-phase generator to produce the x-rays and a multiformat image retrieval system that will include conventional x-ray films as well as television images, movies (cine), and videotape. Most examinations will probably be performed using a combination of several modalities.

Each modality will be described in turn by considering the sequence of a typical examination. First the technologist obtains a preliminary scout film of the abdomen with an overhead x-ray tube. This film is colloquially known as an "overhead," to distinguish it from films the radiologist will later expose, known as "spots." Exposure factors depend on the patient's size and position, but typically the patient receives 100 to 200 mRem gonadal dose and less than 1 rad (1 centigray) skin dose from this single exposure.

The study would continue with the radi-ologist watching on fluoroscopy while the patient is given contrast. With fluoroscopy the radiologist can view the image directly on a television screen without exposing film and waiting for it to be developed; this "real-time" evaluation is especially useful for studying a dynamic, constantly changing system such as the gastrointestinal tract.

Fluoroscopy was made possible by the development of a means whereby x-rays strike a fluorescent screen on which an image can be simultaneously formed and viewed. In early fluoroscopy units, the image was inferior, especially with larger patients, and the examination had to be performed in the dark (always literally, sometimes figuratively!) after the radiologist had first adapted his eyes to the dark by wearing red goggles. With modern equipment, which incorporates an image intensification system, the image can be viewed on a television monitor in comfortably subdued light.

Attached to the image intensification tower is a holder device for cassettes, each cassette containing a film-screen combination. A panel selector allows the radiologist to bring the cassette into the x-ray beam and make a permanent record of what is seen on the TV screen. In addition to conventional ($9\frac{1}{2} \times 9\frac{1}{2}$ or 10×8 in) x-ray film, the system can be adapted for smaller film sizes (70 mm, 100 mm, 105 mm). Areas of interest the radiologist discovers fluoroscopically, and areas not optimally demonstrated on the overhead films, such as the convolutions of the sigmoid colon and the duodenal bulb, are "spot filmed" during the examination. The spot films are not

13

meant to replace or necessarily duplicate the overhead films the technologist takes. Many areas need to be "unfolded" and will be seen well only on adequately positioned spot films. The advantage of this system is that a permanent record can be made when the patient is perfectly positioned; otherwise one runs the risk of missing the abnormality on the overheads, which are exposed according to a set routine.

Since the GI tract is constantly in motion, capturing this action is frequently desirable. Movie cameras (cine) and magnetic tape recorders can be adapted to the basic system; this advance allows a dynamic recording of a dynamic system for later review (and permanent storage if desired).

RADIATION PROTECTION

All people on earth are exposed to an irreducible amount of radiation known as *background radiation*. Since it has never been proved that there is a minimal safe dose of radiation, it is obviously desirable to limit any additional exposure above and beyond the background dose all people get. Unfortunately, medical x-rays account for most of this additional exposure, so it is incumbent upon radiologists to be aware of radiation hazards and to practice radiation protection.

There is considerable debate as to what constitutes a radiation hazard. Some have argued that there is no threshold for radiation damage, and that any amount is potentially harmful in a dose-related way. The problem is further complicated by the fact that radiation effects are considered under two aspects: somatic effects (affecting only the particular individual exposed) and genetic effects (affecting future generations by damage from gonadal exposure). The information regarding these effects is largely derived from statistical projection of scant data, and its reliability has been questioned. Genetic damage from low-dose radiation has not been proved to occur, and respected scientists have recently reversed their opinions on the induction of somatic effects, such as leukemia. In 1980 the

Committee on the Biological Effects of Ionizing Radiation of the National Academy of Sciences finally issued a redraft of a disputed paper on the health risks of low-level radiation. The report scaled down the cancer risk to about half that estimated in 1972. This was accomplished largely by questioning the validity of extrapolating data obtained at high-dose levels (atomic bomb explosions) to low doses. Obviously, not even experts can agree, so presumably the law of parsimony should apply to radiation exposure — in this instance, *less* is better.

Radiation protection is especially important for those at greatest risk: the young and the unborn. The radiologist should assume the responsibility for ensuring that pregnant women are not radiographed (especially during the crucial first trimester), unless absolutely indicated medically. Care should be taken to provide gonadal shielding, especially for children and young adults. In fact, in some states, such as Massachusetts, this is now mandated by law.

There are other ways to further reduce exposure, which should be kept in mind. The number of examinations performed and the number of exposures per examination can be limited by good medical judgment and proper radiographic control (Table 2–1). Even on a given film, exposure can be reduced by careful collimation and the proper choice of film size. The patient is needlessly exposed when the area fluoroscoped or filmed is larger than the area of interest. This applies particularly during fluoroscopy, and the radiologist must continually work the shutters to obtain an appropriate field size at every moment during the examination. Remember these three proscriptions:

1. Don't think with your foot (or finger) on the fluoroscopy switch.

2. Never fluoroscope without using the shutters.

3. Fluoroscope only the area of interest, not the whole patient!

So far, we have discussed ways to decrease exposure to the patient, but exposure to the radiologist and technologist, especially during fluoroscopy, should also be considered. Lead aprons must be worn and do adequately protect the trunk and gonads. The unprotected hands should not be placed in the x-ray beam, as pioneering radiologists found out in their fingerless old age. A lead glove must be worn if it is necessary to manipulate the patient under the intensifier apparatus. Scatter radiation from the patient can be protected against by keeping the intensifier tower as close to the patient as possible; incidentally, this also improves the sharpness of the final image. Since x-ray intensity falls off according to the inverse square law, the farther the radiologist is away from the source, the less exposure he or she gets. Try to avoid hunching over the intensifier. Some advocate lead-glass eyeglasses to protect the lens of the eye from scatter radiation; even regular glasses will cut down lens exposure dramatically.

We have so far put the burden for reducing exposure on the radiologist and technologist, and undoubtedly they can both do much to protect both the patient and themselves by careful attention to detail. Technical improvements, however, can also be utilized to reduce exposure. Reducing fluoroscopic output to the minimum level consistent with good visualization of structures will lower exposure. Many radiologists expose small films, such as 105 mm, instead of conventional spot films; these can provide equal diagnostic accuracy with as little as one tenth the radiation exposure of conventional spot films. One other innovation should be mentioned. "Faster" radiographic screens made with rare earth elements allow an equivalent "photographic" exposure for less radiation exposure, and these have had increasing applicability in many areas of radiology.

TECHNIQUE

What Technique to Use?

There are many techniques available for studying the GI tract, each with specific advantages and disadvantages. Which study is chosen depends on the clinical indication and the condition of the patient. Ideally, the fluoroscopist should know beforehand what he is trying to demonstrate, because this will dictate all future decisions. Does the clinical situation mean that the fluoroscopist must pay special attention to a particular area — e.g., gastroesophageal junction in a patient with heartburn, or the retrogastric area and duodenal C-sweep in a patient with suspected pancreatitis? Which contrast material should be used: regular barium, high-density barium, or water-soluble contrast? Should a single or a double contrast study be performed?

Once you have decided to perform the study, the choice of contrast medium becomes important.

Which Contrast Medium to Use?

Basically the choice breaks down to a barium preparation or Gastrografin (meglumine diatrizoate), a water-soluble contrast medium. Under certain clinical situations, barium is contraindicated and water-soluble contrast is essential; such is the case in *perforation*. Under other circumstances — e.g., suspected *aspiration* — water-soluble contrast is strongly contraindicated and barium is preferable.

TABLE 2–1. ESTIMATED RADIATION EXPOSURE — APPROXIMATE DOSES (mrad)

| Examination | Skin | Gonadal | | Fetus |
		Male	*Female*	
Chest x-ray		<5	<10	
KUB	1000	100–200	200–300	300
Oral cholecystogram		<5	100–200	200
UGI series		100–150	500–600	500–600
Barium Enema		200–1500	800–1000	800
Lumbosacral spine		200–2000	200–700	

Ranges after various sources.

The reasoning behind these choices is sound. Water-soluble contrast (Gastrografin) is rapidly reabsorbed if it leaks and does not pose a hazard in the peritoneal cavity. Barium, on the other hand, is very slowly absorbed (note how long it remains in diverticula after a barium enema), and leakage into the peritoneal cavity has been associated with the development of foreign body granulomas and subsequent adhesions. Gastrografin is extremely hyperosmolar (6 to 10 times the osmolarity of plasma) and will therefore draw fluid toward it; if aspirated into the lung a chemical pulmonary edema will result, which can be fatal. Barium, however, is inert in the lung.

The choice of barium versus water-soluble contrast is less clear in perforations of the esophagus. The classic teaching has been to stay with Gastrografin and then, if no leak is seen, to obtain better detail with a barium swallow. Recently, however, experimental studies have suggested that barium might be preferable in suspected leaks into the mediastinum.

WATER-SOLUBLE CONTRAST MEDIUM.

The mucosal detail obtained with water-soluble contrast material is inferior to that obtained with barium, but it is used in the upper GI tract if searching for a leak or gastric outlet obstruction. Distal to the ligament of Treitz, mucosal detail will be poor owing to rapid dilution (especially if there are increased secretions within the lumen, as in small bowel obstruction) (Fig. 2–1). Water-soluble contrast medium, therefore, is usually not used in the study of the small bowel. In the colon, Gastrografin may be used in suspected diverticulitis if extravasation is especially likely.

BARIUM. There are many different preparations of barium sulfate available, and the profusion of these is confusing to even the initiated, let alone the beginner. So, how does one choose which preparation to use for each study? This depends on what part of the GI tract is to be examined and which technique is to be performed (air versus full-column). Luckily, the manufacturers help to some degree, but there will still be an alarming array of products to choose from.

Many millions of dollars have been spent

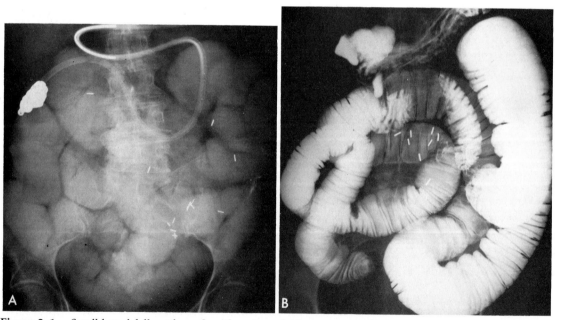

Figure 2–1. *Small bowel follow-through with water-soluble contrast medium. A,* Note how the (meglumine diatrizoate (Gastrografin) rapidly becomes diluted, resulting in very poor mucosal detail. Compare this appearance with a small bowel follow-through with barium as contrast *(B).* The dilated small bowel loops are clearly outlined and obstruction is demonstrated in the midpelvis due to an adhesion.

trying to find the "ideal" barium preparation, but because of the disparate milieux of the esophagus, stomach, small bowel, and colon, different preparations are needed to study different parts of the bowel. Barium that is ideal for an upper GI series will result in a poor air contrast enema, since different properties are needed for the latter.

Basically, for regular UGI and full-column work, a low-density, low-viscosity barium preparation (loosely called "thin" by radiologists), which the x-ray beam can penetrate is required; a denser, somewhat more viscous preparation ("thick") has better *coating* properties for air contrast work.

The "barium" consists of a barium sulfate suspension of a specific particle size with additives to control the charge and absorptive capacity, thus keeping the particles in suspension. An important factor is the density of the preparation and how viscous it is; the higher the viscosity, the slower the flow. The aim is fluidity, with dense, but not excessively viscous, suspensions to improve coating.

The bane of a barium preparation is "flocculation," i.e., the individual barium particles aggregate into clumps, resulting not only in an unesthetic appearance but also in loss of diagnostic information and pseudolesions. Modern barium preparations are designed to stay liquid and not flocculate or clump under physiologic conditions; barium suspensions designed for a small bowel study will stay liquid and in a continuous column (provided enough is given), unless there is an excess of intraluminal fluid, as in malabsorption. Inadequate mixing of barium powder or not shaking the bottle can result in dots that can mimic superficial ulcers. Use of the wrong preparation, such as "regular" barium for an air contrast study, will result not only in poor coating but also in clumping; this is why a

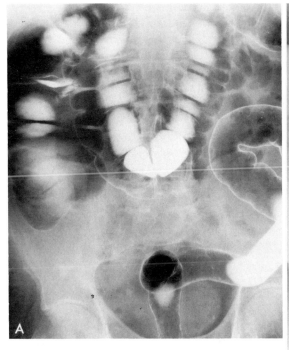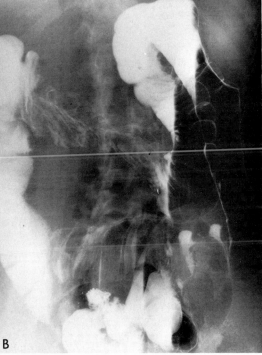

Figure 2–2. *Air contrast enema with poor coating. A,* Note how in the left colon there is adequate, although not ideal, coating; on the right side the colon has not been coated at all. Even large lesions would be missed with this poor coating. This is an inadequate study. *B,* On the decubitus film, the reason for the poor coating is obvious: retained washout fluid. Note how the barium solution is being diluted by the washout in the ascending colon.

full-column enema followed by evacuation in the bathroom and reinsufflation of air is a markedly inferior technique to a primary air contrast examination (Fig. 2–2).

The Choice of Study

One must decide whether a single contrast study is the best one for a particular patient and clinical problem or whether an air contrast study is preferred. The choice between single and double contrast is easier to make for studies of the colon than for the stomach because it has been shown that the double contrast technique is more sensitive in finding polyps. Obviously one does not attempt an air contrast study in a 90 year old patient with a healing fracture of the hip and chronic constipation; one would question whether any study is indicated in that clinical setting. Under certain circumstances, e.g., suspected diverticulitis or suspected obstruction, the full-column technique is definitely preferred. Similarly, the chance of refluxing barium into the terminal ileum or appendix is much higher with the thinner barium used for full-column study than with the dense barium of air contrast; for this reason, the single contrast examination is the study of choice when disease of these areas is suspected. The double-contrast technique demonstrates mucosal detail and therefore is the choice if small lesions, such as those of erosive gastritis, inflammatory bowel disease, polyps, or early carcinoma, are suspected.

An individual decision must be made in each clinical situation concerning which study is more suitable. A single contrast UGI or enema in the hands of an experienced fluoroscopist using adequate compression and pro-file is an excellent technique, although it does have some limitations with smaller lesions. In some situations, it is definitely the procedure of choice. Whichever procedure is chosen, aim to do it well, and remember that an air contrast study with poor coating is as useless as a full-column study without adequate penetration.

Basic Principles of Full-Column Versus Air Contrast Studies (Table 2–2)

SINGLE CONTRAST. In a *single contrast* study, a dilute barium is used to distend the lumen. *Distention* is important, but lesions are primarily seen either by *compression* or by *profile* (two views at right angles are important here). Compression is used to spread the barium column to allow adequate *penetration*, but it is also important to choose the appropriate exposure factors to penetrate the barium column. If the barium preparation is too dense or the kVp (for penetration) too low (average kVp for single contrast UGI series, 110 kV; single contrast enema, 125 kV), lesions will be obscured as neither compression nor penetration will be adequate. It is also important to *"unwind"* any kinks or loops in the bowel; if this is not done, lesions, especially constricting lesions oriented in a plane directed toward the viewer, will be missed. Unwinding is especially important in areas that are difficult if not impossible to compress, such as the flexures.

AIR CONTRAST. *Air contrast* techniques, on the other hand, depend on *coating* the mucosa with a thin layer of dense barium and then *distending* the lumen with air. Although the air contrast study is basically a "see-through" examination, every attempt should still be made to unwind overlapping loops. A lower kilovoltage (90 to 100 kVp) is used to accentuate the contrast between the barium and the air. Films are taken with the patient in different postions; this is done both to unwind loops and to manipulate air and barium into different segments of bowel.

The amount of barium introduced into the colon is vital. Too little barium will result in poor coating and too much will obscure

TABLE 2–2. PRINCIPLES OF SINGLE VERSUS DOUBLE CONTRAST TECHNIQUE

Single Contrast	Air Contrast
Thin barium	Thick barium
Penetration	Coating
Compression	Distention
Profile	See-through
Unwind	Unwind

parts of the bowel, as the preparation is too dense to be penetrated. Similarly, inadequate coating from the wrong barium or as a result of residual washout fluid will cause lesions to be missed. The colon must be adequately distended; otherwise, nonpliable areas in the wall may be missed; at the same time, adequate distention helps to separate or distinguish real pathology from pseudolesions.

Although you may have concluded that the air contrast technique is uniformly superior, it does have its limitations. Certainly a double contrast enema takes longer than a full-column study, and the patient must be mobile and able to cooperate. Use of glucagon aids in distention and is helpful in both the upper and lower studies; the dose required to induce hypotonia is much less for the stomach than for the colon (average, 0.1 to 0.25 mg intravenous injection for stomach, 0.5 to 1.0 mg for the colon).

An attempt will be made to illustrate basic guidelines by considering a routine examination.

Study of the Nonemergency Patient

Some preparation is required for most contrast studies of the gastrointestinal tract, e.g., the patient should be fasting for a UGI or small bowel follow-through since food or liquid (even a cup of coffee) not only will interfere with coating but also may result in pseudolesions. Even antacids may be a problem in this regard and should be withheld for at least 4 hours before the study (a factor commonly overlooked when the patient is told not to eat or drink). If only the esophagus is to be studied (a pure barium swallow), fasting is not necessary.

For a barium enema, a "clean colon" is

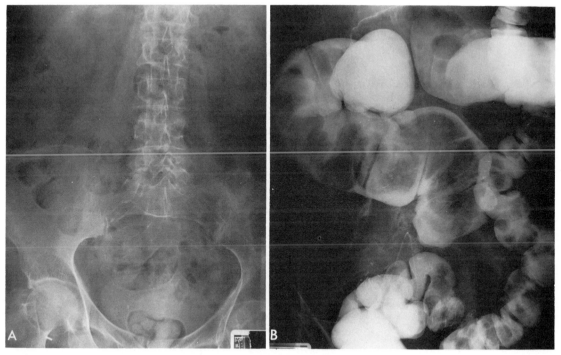

Figure 2–3. *A, Value of the scout film.* A plain abdominal (KUB) film shows a large amount of stool in the right colon and rectum despite oral laxatives and a liquid diet. The preparation was repeated, and the examination was able to be performed the next day (with an empty ["clean"] colon). *B, "Fecogram."* This film shows the result if one were to go ahead with the study in an unprepared patient. Note the large filling defects within the lumen due to feces, any one of which defects could be obscuring a lesion. This study must be repeated after more intensive bowel preparation.

required, and both oral laxatives and a liquid (nonresidue) diet are necessary to rid the colon of its fecal contents; in many institutions, a cleansing enema is added to this regimen. An unprepared colon not only will result in an esthetically displeasing study but also may obscure lesions, since all the filling defects will be assumed to be feces (Fig. 2–3). It has been estimated, for example, that one in five cancers of the colon are missed on initial barium enemas, not because they are not seen, but because they are dismissed as feces. Good bowel preparation is therefore essential. Ideally, it should be the responsibility of the radiologist to ensure this; at the very least he makes the final decision whether to go ahead with the enema or reprepare the patient.

Performing the Studies

There are probably as many ways to perform barium studies as there are radiologists. No attempt, therefore, will be made in this book to instruct the reader *how* to perform exactly each step of a particular study. Rather, basic principles will be stressed, from which an idealized study can be constructed. A table has been included that will provide some basic "cookbook" guidance.

Barium Swallow (BaSw)

Often the patient will be able to pinpoint accurately the level at which dysphagia or food sticking occurs; sometimes, however, this level is referred.

Pharyngeal motility is so swift that rapid sequence cine filming is necessary to study this area adequately. If cine is not available, static studies may be obtained on 70 mm, 100 mm, or 105 mm film (up to 6 frames per sec), or "timed swallows" may be done on spot films, if the patient is cooperative, by exposing the film as the "Adam's apple" reaches its maximal elevation. At this point, the bolus is passing through the pharynx and upper esophagus and will show these areas distend-

ed with barium. Views with the pharynx distended with barium, and then coated with barium and distended with air, are taken in both frontal and lateral projections. A "puffed-cheek" view is necessary to see that the pyriform sinuses distend and are symmetrical. Fluoroscopy of the vocal cords is part of the examination of the pharynx.

The remainder of the esophagus can be studied in many ways, but three factors are important: (1) *peristalsis* must be observed with the patient horizontal (see Chapter 4); (2) look for a hiatus hernia; (3) search for any lesions; two projections at right angles are necessary if a single contrast barium swallow is to be interpreted (a lesion may be detected only on profile if penetration is not adequate). With air contrast, only one view may suffice since this is a "see-through" study.

Upper Gastrointestinal Series (UGI)

A basic principle of any gastrointestinal study is the use of gravity to make the barium and air go into different parts of the organ; since barium is heavy it will sink; air will rise. Each area should be shown filled with barium as the distending agent, or coated with barium and distended with air. To this end, the patient is placed in different positions to allow different parts of the stomach to be visualized.

Although the order in which spot films are taken may vary from patient to patient, certain areas of the stomach and duodenum should always be covered on spot films. The following is a guideline.

Single Contrast UGI Series

Remember that the salient features are *compression, profile*, and *distention*.

1. Compression views of the stomach show fold pattern and pliability (Fig. 2–4).

2. Schatzki view with patient slightly right side down, shows the anterior and posterior wall of the body of the stomach.

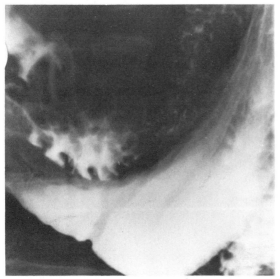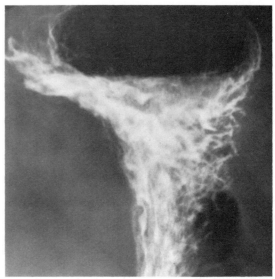

Figure 2–4. *Compression views of the stomach.* A four-on-one spot film is taken, compressing the four quadrants of the stomach, to be able to see that the folds are normal and that there are no filling defects. Two of the spot films are shown.

3. In drinking esophagus view, patient lies prone over a bolster to show peristalsis and hernia.

4. Compression-filled duodenal bulb: The patient should be prone over bolster or erect — whichever way it is done it is necessary to see the folds (Fig. 2–5).

5. Air views of bulb (and distal antrum): The patient is supine with the left side down to make air rise into the antrum (Fig. 2–8) and bulb.

Air Contrast UGI Study

Remember that the objects are *coating* and *distention*. No more than a few ounces of dense barium is given to coat the mucosa; gas is given to distend the stomach, along with an antifoaming agent to prevent bubbles. There are many ways to get gas into the stomach: commercial tablets, powder, or granules that release carbon dioxide are the most common agents; even cola beverages have been used. Routine use of glucagon (0.1 to 0.25 mg intravenous injection) will allow more time to study the stomach and also aids in distention.

An air esophagram can be done simply by getting the patient, who has already been given gas, to gulp the barium rapidly. Make sure gas is not inadvertently given above a stricture — check for dysphagia beforehand. Then concentrate on the stomach.

More time is spent at this point coating and distending the stomach by turning the patient. The aim is to study the stomach before letting barium dump into the duodenum. For this reason, the patient is turned prone over his *left* side and back to the supine position when coating the stomach. Four or five spot films of the stomach are taken once there is adequate coating.

A sample routine could be as follows:

1. Give glucagon intravenously.

2. Administer gas powder and water with a few drops of Mylicon.

3. Have the patient gulp barium; take erect air views of esophagus.

4. Supine stomach view (for body). Turn the patient prone to coat anterior wall of the stomach, then *left* side down to coat greater curvature, then supine (Fig. 2–7.) At this stage, the lesser curvature may not be coated and it may be necessary to turn the patient right side down to coat it (if the patient is turned slowly

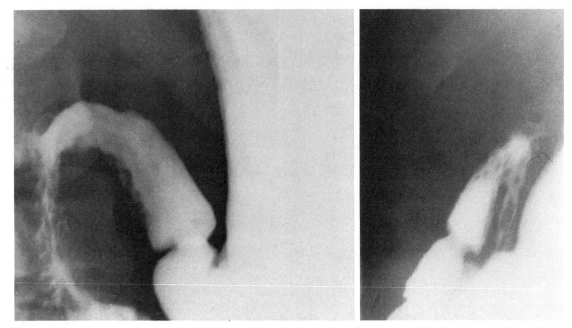

Figure 2–5. *Compression views of duodenal bulb.* A normal triangular duodenal bulb unwound from the C-sweep is seen on the left. On the right is the opposite profile at 90 degrees (patient is now turned from lying on his right side toward the supine position until the duodenal bulb peeps out from behind the stomach).

to the right and quickly back left again, dumping of barium into the duodenum is less likely to occur).

5. Place patient left side down for view of antrum; wait until it empties of barium and fills with air.

6. Right lateral view. Make sure all the barium has run out of the fundus so the gastroesophageal junction can be seen en face; this is the only time you will see it in air — make sure the anterior wall is also visible filled.

7. Prone, perhaps semierect view. This is a good view for the air-filled fundus (although if the stomach is horizontal, an erect view may give a better fundal picture). At the same time, compression by bolster should show the folds in the antrum.

8. Take prone esophagus view as for single contrast examination.

9. Take filled compressed duodenal bulb view as for single contrast examination.

10. Take air-filled antrum, duodenal bulb, and C-sweep views as for single contrast examination (Fig. 2–8).

A standard set of overhead films has been worked out, which allows not only another look at the esophagus, stomach, and duodenum, but also shows the relationship of these to surrounding structures (Fig. 2–6). Table 2–3 will help to clarify why different overhead views are necessary and what is best visualized in each one.

The Barium Enema

Gravity is especially important in helping the barium to flow through the colon during an enema; appropriate use of gravity will permit the use of less barium, and there will be less discomfort for the patient. Spot films are taken of certain areas that are difficult to see on the overhead films owing to overlapping.

In certain parts of the colon, if the x-ray beam is perpendicular to the film and the patient, loops of bowel oriented directly toward or away from the beam are overlapped and foreshortened. Lesions in these loops may therefore be missed. These loops can be elon-

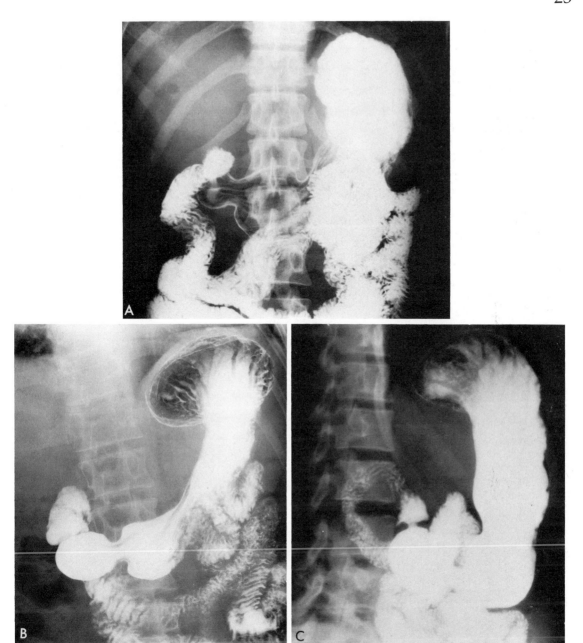

Figure 2–6. *Overhead films from "regular" UGI. A,* Supine film shows the air-filled antrum with the fundus filled with barium. *B,* Prone film; note how this is basically a mirror image of *A. C,* A right-side-down prone oblique view gives a very good picture of the duodenum bulb and C-sweep and also the lesser curvature. Not illustrated is a right lateral stomach.

gated and "unwound" by turning the patient into an oblique position or by angling the x-ray tube, or both; the beam will then be directed along the loop of bowel. This is especially useful in the sigmoid colon (there is even a view called the Chassard-Lapiné view, for which the patient has to sit upright on the enema tip). Decubitus views are essential in the air contrast enema because the barium and air layer onto different sides of the loops; indeed, it has been said that these are the most useful films in the whole examination.

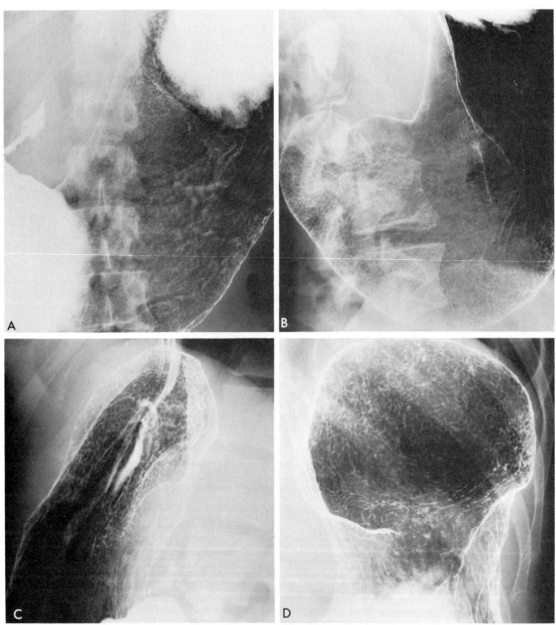

Figure 2–7. *Normal air contrast upper GI series. A, A supine* film demonstrates barium in both the fundus and antrum of the stomach. The body is well distended and the areae gastricae are nicely outlined. *B,* With the patient turned slightly *left side down,* air now bubbles up into the antrum, which is well distended and coated, showing normal areae. *C,* A *right lateral* view shows the fundus of the stomach well distended with air and the anterior and posterior walls of the stomach clearly defined. The gastroesophageal rosette in this case is more like a hood. The white line on the posterior wall of the stomach is an extrinsic pressure defect from a normal pancreas. *D, Prone view of stomach.* In this position the fundus will fill with air. Some compression of the body can be obtained by placing a bolster underneath the abdomen so that the fold pattern can be seen. Note that this film is printed in the anatomic position rather than as one would see it fluoroscopically.

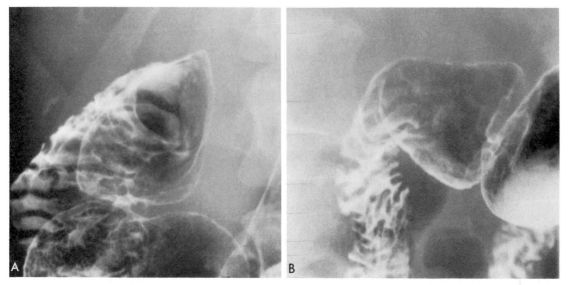

Figure 2–8. *A, Air-filled duodenal bulb.* Although the duodenal bulb is well distended with air, technique is not adequate, as the bulb has not been swung off the C-sweep. Compare this with a subsequent film *(B)*, when the patient has been turned more to the left; this allows an unimpeded view of the duodenal bulb without overlap from the descending C-sweep and would allow an ulcer at the apex of the bulb to be seen.

TABLE 2–3.   OVERHEADS GIVE THE BIG PICTURE

Examination	Overhead Film	Especially Useful For
Single contrast UGI series	Prone right anterior oblique (drinking esophagus view) Right anterior oblique stomach Right lateral stomach Prone KUB Supine KUB	Mass effect upon esophagus Mass effect on duodenal bulb and C-sweep Mass displacing stomach.
Double contrast UGI series	Many believe that no overhead films are necessary, but if obtained, a similar set to that for single contrast will suffice	
Single contrast enema	Prone Supine Lateral rectum Prone angled rectosigmoid ⎫ Supine angled oblique sigmoid ⎭ Oblique prone and supine abdomen as required	Measurement of presacral space Unwinding and stretching of sigmoid
Double contrast enema	Prone Supine Prone cross-table rectum Right and left lateral decubitus Prone angled rectosigmoid ⎫ Supine angled oblique sigmoid ⎭ Supine and/or prone oblique if colon is extremely redundant	Rectal mucosa Whole colon—these are vital! Unwinding of sigmoid

The Full-Column Enema

Again, *compression, profile,* and *distention* are the key words. The purpose of this technique is to spot-film areas that will not be displayed to advantage on the overhead films, although *all* areas of the colon should be observed fluoroscopically (Fig. 2–9). An example of spot filming technique would be as follows:

1. Left lateral rectum view; start with the patient lying on left side.

2. Oblique view(s) of the sigmoid colon. By turning the patient slowly toward and partly onto his back as you watch on fluoroscopy, the sigmoid colon can be seen to elongate and unwind; if it has multiple convolutions more than one spot film in different obliquities will be needed.

3. Splenic flexure view. Turn the patient onto his *right side* until the flexure is unfolded.

Incidentally, in this position, gravity will aid in filling the transverse colon.

4. Hepatic flexure view. Turn the patient toward the opposite side to unfold this flexure.

5. Compression views of the cecum. Make sure the ileocecal valve, terminal ileum, or appendix are seen before you are satisfied that you have filled the whole cecum and are not overlooking something.

6. Don't forget to palpate the whole colon, either with a lead-gloved hand, a paddle, or a compression cone looking for filling defects.

Double Contrast Enema

There are many variations on this newer technique, and even among experts, there is disagreement about many aspects, such as

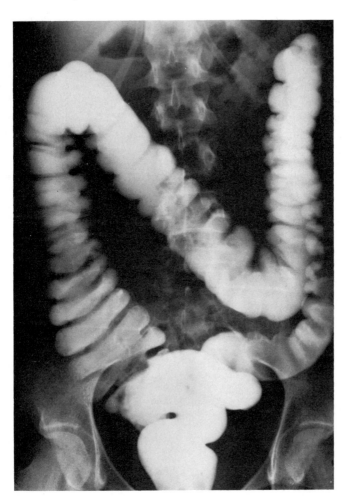

Figure 2–9. *Supine film from a full column enema.* There is moderately good distention of the whole colon, and good penetration has been obtained. Note, however, that this single view is inadequate for the study of the sigmoid colon, and although in this patient the hepatic flexure is reasonably well displayed, the splenic flexure is overlapped.

when the colon should be drained and the order and timing of spot films.

Fluoroscopy is especially important to maneuver the *correct* amount of barium around the colon (Fig. 2–10).

1. With the patient prone (to aid flow of heavy barium into sigmoid), advance the barium to the splenic flexure.

2. At this point, the object is to run in only enough barium to coat the transverse and right colon without flooding them. This may be done either purely by gravity (patient lying with his right side down) or by a combination of gravity and air insufflation. It is vital to keep air from getting ahead of the advancing barium column; this can be prevented by keeping the barium column dependent so that it moves as a bolus.

3. Once sufficient barium has reached the hepatic flexure, excess may be drained from the left colon by bringing the patient upright. If there is too much barium in the right colon (an error in judgment — too much barium was allowed to run in), this position may result in reflux. For this reason, some advocate taking spot films of the sigmoid early.

4. As you continue to insufflate air, spot films of the following must be taken: (a) rectum (prone following drainage), (b) sigmoid colon, (c) flexures (erect), (d) transverse colon (erect), (e) cecum.

5. *Overhead films* are particularly important in the air contrast enema. Proper radiographic technique is vital.

"PROBLEM PATIENTS"

It is easy to obtain good studies of the fit patient. Problems arise when patients are too

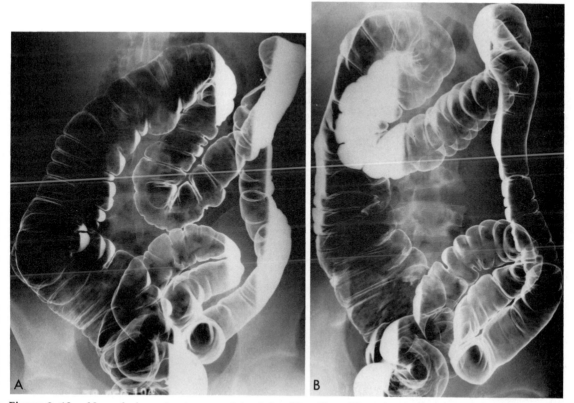

Figure 2–10. *Normal air contrast enema, lateral decubitus films.* There is excellent coating and distention with an adequate but not excessive amount of barium layering. Note how these mirror-image pictures allow you to see half the colon on each film.

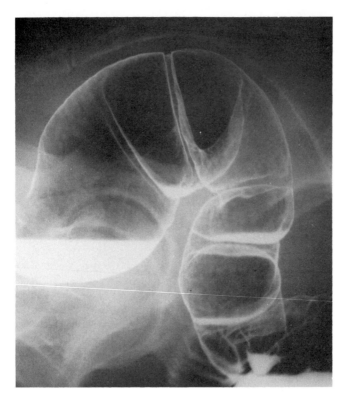

Figure 2–11. *Prone cross-table rectum.* This film is taken following drainage of the rectum in the prone position. This view allows excellent visualization of almost all of the rectal mucosa and is especially useful in searching for polyps on the valves of Houston. Note how narrow the presacral space is.

Figure 2–12. *Prone angled rectosigmoid.* With the patient prone and the tube angled 30 to 35 degrees caudad (towards the feet) the sigmoid is elongated and there is less overlap. The rectum, however, is foreshortened, and this is not a view to use for observing the distal rectum. Note that there is a polyp in the proximal sigmoid (arrow) and multiple diverticula. Although a small amount of contrast medium and air has refluxed into the terminal ileum, this is not interfering with interpretation of the sigmoid.

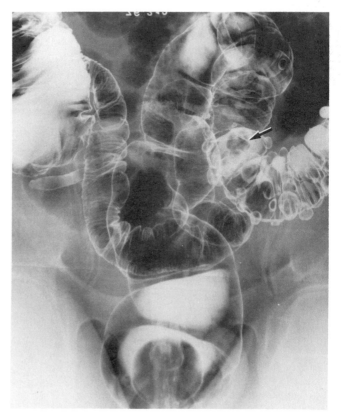

sick to move or cooperate fully. The following are some short cuts and hints which may come in handy with these patients.

The Extremely Ill Patient (The Supine, Gravity-Aided Upper GI Study)

In the patient who is too weak to move or who is in severe pain, gravity must be utilized to the fullest to maneuver barium and air within the stomach into the positions necessary to demonstrate the anatomy. To save the patient unnecessary effort and the radiologist's and technologist's backs, as few movements as possible should be used in this study. It is possible to obtain quite a respectable study in this way even in a patient who has to be maneuvered bodily (but gently) into the various positions.

A simple method is as follows:

1. With the patient partly on the right side, drinking esophagus and Schatzki views are taken.

2. With patient lying on right side and slightly prone, the duodenal bulb and C-sweep will then be filled with barium.

3. Turn the patient gradually onto his back; compression spot films of different areas of the stomach are taken as he turns.

4. With the patient halfway onto his left side, air views of the distal antrum, duodenal bulb, and C-sweep are obtained. If the patient is extremely ill, cannot sit up, or is nauseated, he may not be able to swallow (and keep down) gas, pills, or powder. Air may then be introduced into the stomach by putting an additional hole in the straw with a needle; as a result, every time the patient drinks, not only barium but also air will be swallowed, thus distending the stomach.

5. Regular overhead films may then be made by the technologist after the patient has been given additional barium to drink.

In the description just given, patient movement is minimized to gain maximum information. Most patients can in fact perform these few movements with some assistance if they are constantly encouraged during the examination. It is important to understand that if the patient cannot turn prone, lesions on the anterior wall may be missed.

The Patient Who Cannot or Will Not Drink the Barium

In this case, the essential thing is to make sure that the examination is critical to the patient's care. If the examination is vital, two approaches may be taken. Some patients who will not swallow from either a cup or through a straw will do so if a catheter-tip syringe is put into the corner of the mouth and the barium is slowly injected. This may be especially useful in the mentally retarded patient. One must, however, be careful not to overfill the patient's mouth since then there is the risk of aspiration. Another approach is to introduce a nasogastric tube into the stomach (either in the radiology department or before the patient is brought there). Barium and air can then be introduced at will; by positioning the patient appropriately, an adequate study can be obtained.

The Patient Unable to Retain the Enema

There are a number of situations in which the patient is unable to "hold onto" the barium. Loss of anal tone may be overcome in many patients by inflating the balloon of a balloon catheter; the balloon thus occludes the rectal ampulla. Air should be introduced into the balloon under fluoroscopy, but *the balloon should never be inflated if rectal disease is suspected* (Fig. 2–13). *Spasm,* commonest in the sigmoid colon, may occur. Glucagon given intravenously (in a dose of 0.5 to 1 mg) will help by relaxing the spasm and thus will allow the examination to continue. It is risking the prospect of barium all over the table to continue to run in more barium or contrast if there is persistent spasm; patience is required and one should wait until the spasm has relaxed before proceeding. By the same token, an obstructing lesion that will not allow barium to pass through will result in the patient's "losing the enema." This should be carefully sought for whenever there is unexplained inability to retain the barium before just giving up on the study.

If there is neither spasm nor obstruction, and glucagon has been given, continuing in-

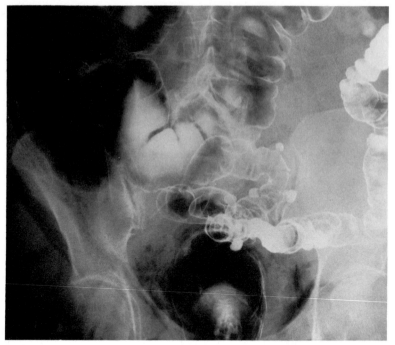

Figure 2–13. *Rectal perforation during barium enema.* An air contrast study with poor mucosal coating demonstrates multiple diverticula and a small polyp in the sigmoid. Look carefully, however, as there is also extravasation of air into the pelvic soft tissues; air is dissecting along the muscle bundles into the thigh and along the muscles of the anterior abdominal wall. The rectal tube has abraded the anterior rectal wall and perforated it. Luckily the perforation was extraperitoneal and no serious sequelae resulted.

Figure 2–14. *Peroral pneumocolon.* A decubitus film from an "air contrast enema" performed following oral administration of sorbitol-containing barium. Following rectal insufflation of air, quite a reasonable study of the right colon can be obtained by this method, although there is interference from overlying small bowel. One large and two small polyps (arrows) are demonstrated in the ascending colon; these were the cause of the patient's GI blood loss.

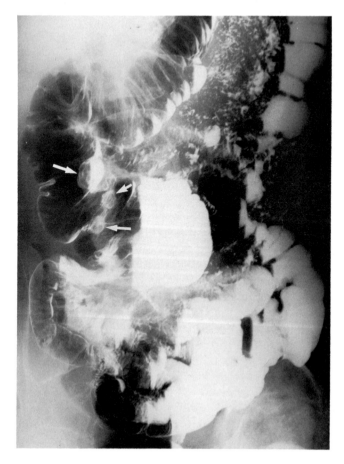

ability to "hang on" is presumably due to loss of anal tone. Taping the buttocks together, holding the enema tip in place with a lead-gloved hand, and putting the table into the Trendelenburg position may help. Sometimes a patient can "hold" in the prone position better than in the lateral or supine position. In patients having difficulty retaining the barium, it is extremely important not only to take spot films as quickly and rapidly as possible but also to run the barium in at a steady pace so as not to overdistend the rectum. One may either "spot as one goes," adding spot films of the descending and transverse colon to the routine spot films, thus covering the whole colon on spot films, or run the contrast medium rapidly to the cecum to make sure that there is no obstructing lesion and then take spot films very quickly of the whole colon. Again, one must use gravity to the fullest as an aid during the study; for example, the patient is turned on his right side to fill the transverse colon and back to the supine position to get the barium around the hepatic flexure.

In general, with these patients the overhead films will not be as contributory as spot films; the time involved in taking them will usually result in the patient losing the enema.

If only the left colon can be examined retrogradely we can study the right colon by the ingenious "barium cocktail" (peroral pneumocolon) in which oral barium is given mixed with sorbitol to make it travel faster through to the colon (Fig. 2–14). When this reaches the right colon, quite a reasonable study of this area can be obtained following administration of intravenous glucagon and rectal insufflation of air.

PITFALLS IN TECHNIQUE — HINTS TO OVERCOME SOME COMMON PROBLEMS

There are a number of problems that may arise during gastrointestinal examinations, and one should know how to cope with these. The following are some of the more common:

POOR COATING (OR POOR DISTENTION). Double-contrast coating will be poor if there is too much fluid relative to the amount of barium. Addition of more barium or rolling the patient may result in better coating as more barium is washed across the surface of the mucosa. Sometimes, however, good coating can never be obtained — e.g., if there is a huge volume of fluid in the stomach. Here the decision should be made to abort the double-contrast study and convert to single contrast. Under these circumstances, simply ask the patient to belch up the gas (this will occur naturally if the patient is brought erect) and start the study again with erect compression views. Continue with a single-contrast study (remember to tell the technologist to increase the kVp for adequate penetration).

Poor coating of the mucosa will result in lesions being missed. To salvage a poor air contrast study, compression films are necessary at the end of the examination if adequate coating has not been obtained, or if on the prone film mucosal folds cannot be seen.

Poor distention is equally bad; if the patient belches or gas escapes rapidly into the duodenum, more gas may be given, but, if there is still not adequate distention, it is better to convert to a single-contrast examination (the same is true if the patient cannot hold the air in during an air contrast enema; lack of distention will obscure even large lesions).

Remember that if in doubt the best policy is *abort and convert* — a poor air contrast study is worse than useless (Fig. 2–15).

CANNOT GET VIEWS OF AIR-FILLED DUODENAL BULB. This is especially likely to occur during the performance of an air contrast study, as overdistention of the stomach pushes the duodenal bulb into a posterior position. The true lateral position will often be best for both filled and air views. In some cases, the bulb may be seen through the air-filled antrum or may be swung anterior to the stomach. Continue to turn the patient from the left lateral position further forward onto his stomach over a bolster; the bolster is needed to prevent barium from running down into the antrum. At the same time, an air-filled view of the anterior wall of the stomach can be obtained (a routine view in Japan).

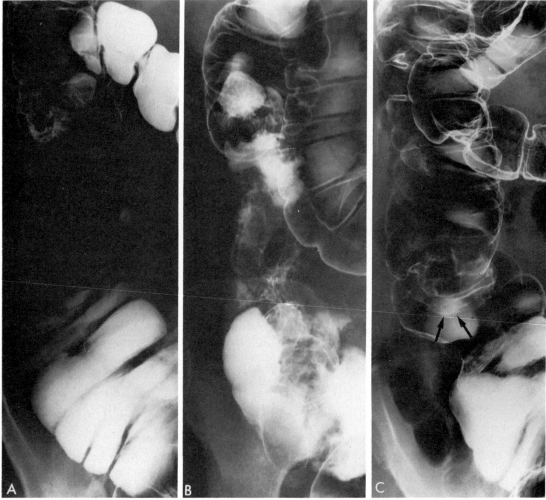

Figure 2–15. *Distention and exposure factors are vital in air contrast enemas. A,* An overpenetrated, overexposed film does not adequately examine the ascending colon. *B,* On another film, this same area is underdistended and even large lesions could be missed. *C,* A repeat film after more air insufflation and with proper radiographic technique demonstrates a large polypoidal cancer (arrows) in the mid-ascending colon.

RAPID EMPTYING INTO THE DUODEN-UM. This problem has been partly solved by using glucagon; many radiologists use it routinely in air contrast work. With glucagon, gastric emptying is slowed and better distention is obtained. In a few patients, despite administration of glucagon, barium will empty rapidly into the duodenum. In these cases, one must *immediately* take air views of the antrum and body before they are covered by the duodenal C-sweep; multiple spots in varying obliquities may be necessary. There is no hurry to get views of the fundus, since one can always come back to it later. Once the body and antrum are covered by loops of small bowel, however, these areas are lost irrevocably to adequate study.

TOO MUCH BARIUM IN THE COLON ON AIR CONTRAST. If there is too much barium relative to the amount of air, some of the colon may not be seen in air contrast, despite multiple views (Fig. 2–16). If you think that there is too much barium, first take the lateral decubitus pictures; if on these more than half of the width of the lumen is filled with barium, too much contrast has been given. At this stage,

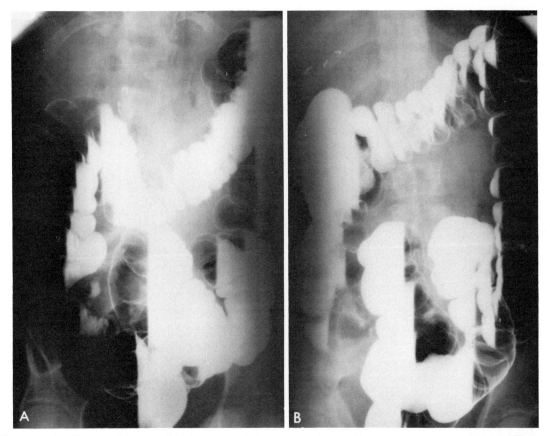

Figure 2–16. *Too much barium.* Much too much barium has been allowed to run into the colon, resulting in most of the colon being obscured by the dense preparation rather than coated with barium but distended with air. Compare this appearance with the decubitus views in Figure 2–10.

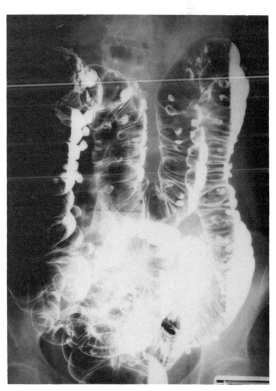

Figure 2–17. *Massive reflux into the distal small bowel.* With such a large amount of reflux as this, the sigmoid colon cannot be seen at all owing to the overlapping of contrast-filled loops of small bowel. One can guard against this by taking spot films of the sigmoid early and keeping the patient prone (do the supine overhead film last).

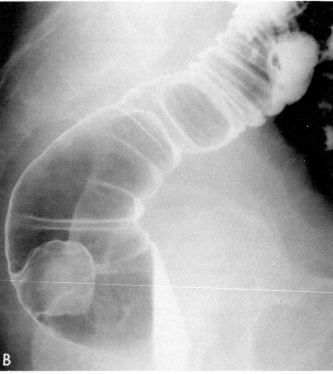

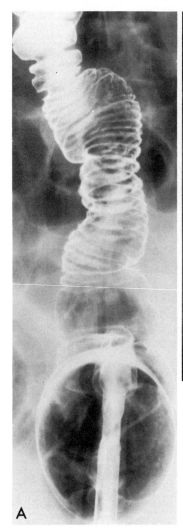

Figure 2–18. *Deflate the balloon; otherwise rectal lesions will be missed.* A, Air contrast enema with the rectal balloon markedly inflated does not show any evidence of a lesion within the rectum; note, however, how much of the rectum is obscured by the balloon. B, A cross-table film of the rectum with the balloon deflated shows a large polypoid lesion. Despite its size, this was a benign villous adenoma. (Courtesy of Ervin Philipps, M.D., Tufts New England Medical School, Boston, Massachusetts.)

oblique films may help, or the patient may be told to evacuate (hoping that this will get rid of both air and barium). The tip is then reinserted and more air is insufflated; this naturally should be done quickly or the barium may cake.

Barium Refluxing Into the Terminal Ileum During an Air Enema. This is a disaster because barium in the small bowel will overlie the sigmoid colon and results in an unreadable confusion of overlapping loops (Fig. 2–17). If barium does reflux, the patient should be put immediately into the prone position; in this position, the ileocecal valve is facing up, so that, it is hoped, only air and not barium will reflux. As an added

precaution, the prone overhead films may be taken first, then the decubitus films, with the supine films last.

PITFALLS IN INTERPRETATION

Poor studies will result in poor diagnosis. There are, however, a number of problems particularly associated with the interpretation of air contrast studies.

Barium artifacts should not be confused with real lesions; this is especially important in the colon where mucous and slime may cause flocculation of the barium, especially with a prolonged examination. Even under

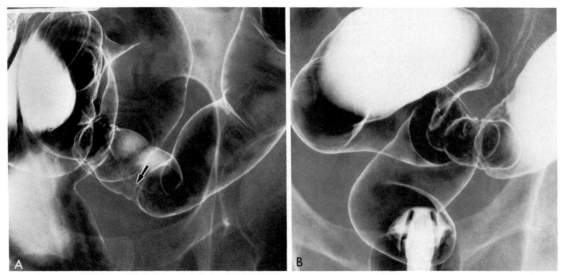

Figure 2–19. *A, Extra lines do not belong.* In the film of the sigmoid colon, if you match up the opposite walls, there is a line (arrow) that does not belong — what might this represent? *B,* An oblique view with the patient turned somewhat more to the left and the sigmoid colon more unwound shows that the extra line within the air column is due to the edge of a carcinoma. The irregular outlines of the carcinoma can now be seen on the superior surface of the sigmoid colon.

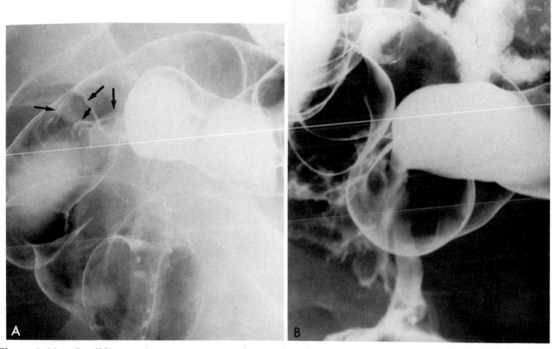

Figure 2–20. *Small lines and crescents do not belong within the air column.* A, On the lateral rectal view there are a number of intersecting white lines just below the rectosigmoid junction (arrows). *B,* A film at 90 degrees shows that these represent the edges of a very large applecore-type lesion.

ideal conditions, an occasional batch of barium may not be fully suspended, resulting in dense white dots. This may occur in both the stomach and the colon; these white dots should not be confused with erosions or aphthoid ulcers.

Occasionally one may not be able to unwind all loops because of the marked distention, but one relies on the "see-through" effect and may not have the benefit of profiling. Even a large lesion may appear only as a number of lines or even a single line when seen en face. Quite large lesions, such as polyps or cancers, may be represented by quite small lines (Fig. 2–19). Special attention should be paid to any added *lines* or *crescents* within the column of air (Fig. 2–20).

Even if a loop cannot be unwound, an attempt should be made to match the contours of the opposite walls; any extra lines do not belong and may represent the edge of a lesion. Failure to pay attention to added lines has given the air contrast method a bad name because some very large lesions can be overlooked unless there is meticulous attention to such details. Crescents are also a useful sign and should be searched for carefully, since they may represent either partially coated polyps or partially filled ulcer craters. Remember that nothing should be seen within the air column apart from normal rugae and haustra and the normal surface markings of the bowel (areae gastricae or innominate grooves).

APPENDIX A–1. SPOT FILMS FOR SINGLE CONTRAST UGI

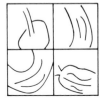

MUCOSAL VIEWS OF
STOMACH (ERECT
COMPRESSION)

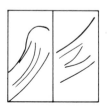

SCHATZKI'S —
SUPINE, RIGHT
SIDE DOWN

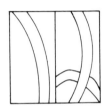

DRINKING ESOPHAGUS
PRONE, RIGHT SIDE
DOWN

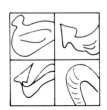

EN FACE ANTRUM

EN FACE BULB   PRONE OR ERECT

PROFILE BULB   COMPRESSION

EN FACE C-SWEEP

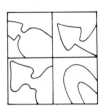

AIR-FILLED ANTRUM   SUPINE, LEFT SIDE DOWN

AIR-FILLED BULB

AIR-FILLED BULB

AIR-FILLED C-SWEEP

APPENDIX A–2. SPOT FILMS FOR AIR CONTRAST UGI

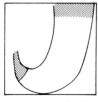

SUPINE (BODY)

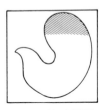

ANTRUM (LEFT SIDE DOWN)

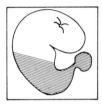

RIGHT LATERAL (GASTROESOPHAGEAL JUNCTION AND ANTERIOR WALL)

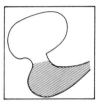

PRONE AND/OR ERECT (FUNDUS)

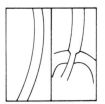

ESOPHAGUS, THEN GE JUNCTION (PRONE OBLIQUE)

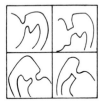

FILLED BULB AND C-SWEEP (PRONE OBLIQUE) WITH COMPRESSION, AND AIR BULB AND C-SWEEP (SUPINE OBLIQUE)

OPTIONAL: Anterior wall views in air contrast.

APPENDIX A–3. SPOT FILMS FOR FULL COLUMN ENEMA

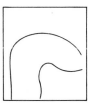

LEFT LATERAL RECTUM

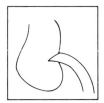

OBLIQUE SIGMOID,
LEFT SIDE DOWN

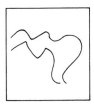

OBLIQUE SIGMOID
(PRONE)

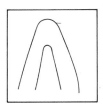

SPLENIC FLEXURE,
RIGHT SIDE DOWN

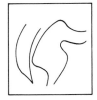

HEPATIC FLEXURE,
LEFT SIDE DOWN

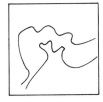

CECUM (SUPINE WITH
COMPRESSION)

At the end of the spot films, the entire colon is palpated
with the lead-gloved hand.

APPENDIX A–4. SPOT FILMS FOR AIR CONTRAST ENEMA

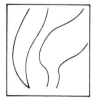

LATERAL RECTUM
(AND/OR PRONE
RECTUM)

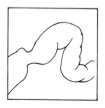

OBLIQUE SIGMOID

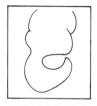

CECUM (SUPINE)

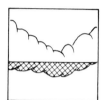

TRANSVERSE COLON
(ERECT)

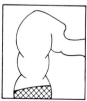

HEPATIC FLEXURE
(ERECT)

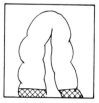

SPLENIC FLEXURE
(ERECT)

APPENDIX A–5.

SUPINE   PRONE

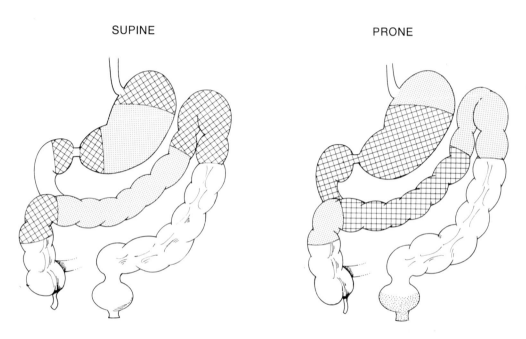

Supine and prone films are the mirror image of each other—if a loop is filled with barium in one position, to fill it with air, merely turn the patient over.

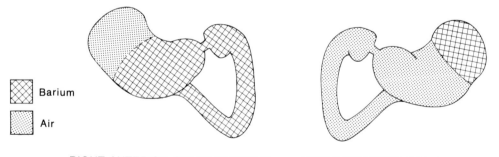

▨	Barium
▨	Air

RIGHT ANTERIOR OBLIQUE PRONE   LEFT POSTERIOR OBLIQUE SUPINE

References

General

Miller RE, Skucas J: Radiographic Contrast Agents. Baltimore, University Park Press, 1977.

Radiation Technology

Brent RL, Gorson RO: Radiation exposure in pregnancy. Curr Probl Radiol 2:5, 1972.

Casarett GW: Possible effects of relatively low levels of radiation. Curr Probl Radiol 3:2, 1973.

Christensen EE, Curry TS III, Dowdey JE: An Introduction to the Physics of Diagnostic Radiology. Philadelphia, Lea & Febiger, 1978.

Coggle JE: Biological Effects of Radiation. New York, Springer-Verlag, 1971.

Fabrikant JI: Radiobiology. Chicago, Year Book Medical Publishers, 1972.

Hall EJ: Radiobiology for the Radiologist. New York, Harper & Row, 1973.

Land CE: Estimating cancer risks from low doses of ionizing radiation. Science 209:1197–1203, 1980.

National Research Council, Advisory Committee on the Biological Effects of Ionizing Radiations: The Effects on Populations of Exposure to Low Levels of Ionizing Radiation. Washington, DC, National Academy of Sciences, 1980.

Schulz RJ: Diagnostic X-ray Physics. New York, GAF Corporation, 1977.

Selman J: The Fundamentals of X-ray and Radium Physics. Springfield, Ill., Charles C Thomas, 1972.

Esophagus

Cockerill EM, Miller RE, Chernish SM, McLaughlin GC III, Rodda BE: Optimal visualization of esophageal varices. Am J Roentgenol 126:512, 1976.

Goldstein HM, Dodd GD: Double-contrast examination of the esophagus. Gastrointest Radiol 1:2, 1976.

Skucas J, Schrank WW: The routine air-contrast examination of the esophagus. Radiology 115:482–484, 1975.

Stomach

Gelfand DW: The Japanese-style double-contrast examination of the stomach. Gastrointest Radiol 1:7, 1976.

Goldsmith MR, Paul RE Jr, Poplack WE, Moore JP, Matsue H, Bloom S: Evaluation of routine double contrast views of the anterior wall of the stomach. Am J Roentgenol 126:1159–1163, 1976.

Laufer I: A simple method for routine double-contrast study of the upper gastrointestinal tract. Radiology 117:513–518, 1975.

Laufer I, Mullens JE, Hamilton J: The diagnostic accuracy of barium studies of the stomach and duodenum — correlation with endoscopy. Radiology 115:596–574, 1975.

Miller RE: The air-contrast stomach examination: an overview. Radiology 117:743–744, 1975.

Poplack W, Paul RE, Goldsmith M, Matsue H, Moore JP, Norton R: Demonstration of erosive gastritis by the double-contrast technique. Radiology 117:519–521, 1975.

Postoperative Stomach

Gohel VK, Laufer I: Double-contrast examination of the postoperative stomach. Radiology 129:601–607, 1978.

Gold RP, Seaman WB: The primary double-contrast examination of the postoperative stomach. Radiology 124:297–305, 1977.

Small Bowel

Ekberg O: Double contrast examination of the small bowel. Gastrointest Radiol 1:349–353, 1977.

Miller RE: Barium sulfate in small bowel examinations. Radiol Clin North Am 7:185–187, 1969.

Miller RE, Sellink JL: Enteroclysis: The small bowel enema. How to succeed and how to fail. Gastrointest Radiol 4:269–284, 1979.

Sanders DE, Ho CS: The small bowel enema: Experience with 150 examinations. Am J Roentgenol 127:743–752, 1976.

Colon

Clayton RS: A clean colon in one hour. Appl Radiol, pp 69–80, Nov-Dec, 1980.

Ettinger A, Elkin M: Study of the sigmoid by special roentgenographic views. Am J Roentgenol 72:199–208, 1954.

Kellett MJ, Zboralske FF, Margulis AR: Per oral pneumocolon examination of the ileocecal region. Gastrointest Radiol 1:361–365, 1977.

Laufer I: The double-contrast enema: Myths and misconceptions. Gastrointest Radiol 1:19–31, 1976.

Miller RE: Examination of the colon. Curr Probl Radiol 5:3–40, 1975.

Ott DJ, Gelfan DW, Wu WC, Kerr RM: Sensitivity of double-contrast barium enema: emphasis on polyp detection. Am J Roentgenol 135:327–330, 1980.

Peterson, GH, Miller RE: The barium enema: a reassessment looking toward perfection. Radiology 128:315–320, 1978.

Pochaczevsky R: Oral examination of the colon: "the colonic cocktail." Am J Roentgenol 121:318–325, 1974.

Stevenson CA: The development of the colon examination. Am J Roentgenol 71:385–397, 1954.

Thoeni RF, Margulis AR: The state of radiographic technique in the examination of the colon: a survey. Radiology 127:317–324, 1978.

Thoeni RF, Menuck L: Comparison of barium enema and colonoscopy in the detection of small colonic polyps. Radiology 124:631–636, 1977.

Pitfalls in Interpretation

Ho CS, Rubin E: Linear shadows in the air-contrast barium enema. Radiology 127:621–625, 1978.

Glucagon and Hypotonic Studies

Carsen GM, Finby N: Hypotonic duodenography with glucagon: a clinical comparison study. Radiology 118:529–534, 1976.

Gohel VK, Dalinka MK, Mandell GA, Azimi F: Pharmacoradiology of the gastrointestinal tract. CRC Crit Rev Clin Radiol Nucl Med 5:69–110, 1974.

Merlo RB, Stone M, Baugus P, Martin M: The use of Pro-banthine to induce gastrointestinal hypotonia. Radiology 127:61–62, 1978.

Miller RE, Chernish SM, Brunelle RL: Gastrointestinal radiography with glucagon. Gastrointest Radiol 4:1–10, 1979.

Miller RE, Chernish SM, Brunelle RL, Rosenak BD: Dose response to intramuscular glucagon during hypotonic radiography. Radiology 127:49–54, 1978.

Miller RE, Chernish SM, Brunelle RL, Rosenak BD: Double-blind radiographic study of dose response to intravenous glucagon for hypotonic duodenography. Radiology 127:55–60, 1978.

Miller RE, Chernish SM, Skucas J, Rosenak BD, Rodda BE: Hypotonic roentgenography with glucagon. Am J Roentgenol 121:264, 1974.

Ominsky SH, Moss AA: The postoperative stomach: a comparative study of double-contrast barium examinations and endoscopy. Gastrointest Radiol 4:17–22, 1979.

Rennell CL: Diagnostic value of hypotonic duodenography. Am J Roentgenol 121:256–263, 1974.

3

THE EMERGENCY PATIENT

This chapter will deal first with the patient with an acute abdomen thought to be due to disease of the GI tract; the patient with suspected abdominal trauma will be discussed separately.

It should be understood that plain films of the abdomen are very difficult to interpret. Often, however, these will give vital information not obtainable on clinical examination, and therefore it is necessary to become expert in their interpretation. Before reading any films, it is extremely important to have as much clinical information as possible, and, to this end, close rapport with the clinician is essential. It is the role of the radiologist not only to help the clinician to come to a diagnosis, but also to look for any *danger signs* indicating the need for immediate treatment, such as closed loop obstruction, ischemic loops, impending gangrene, or perforation. Often the radiologist is the first to suggest that complications indicating the need for immediate operation have set in.

ACUTE ABDOMINAL SERIES

To evaluate the patient with an "acute abdomen," a series of films known as *the acute abdominal series* are taken. It has been shown that there is an optimal sequence of films, taken in different positions that will give the maximum amount of information. This is as follows:

1. Left lateral decubitus (left side to table) abdominal film.
2. Erect chest film.
3. Erect abdominal film.
4. Supine abdominal film.

There is a rationale behind this sequence. The aim of positioning is to allow any "free air" to be maneuvered into a position where it can be readily seen—namely, over the liver (Fig. 3–1). The patient should come to the x-ray department from the emergency room on his left side, which will allow any air in the lesser sac to escape into the general peritoneal cavity and also allow any other free air to rise up over the liver. There is another reason why the left-side-down position is chosen; if the patient were lying on his right side, any free air would rise to lie over the stomach and splenic flexure and would be difficult to see.

Ideally, every effort should be made to obtain both an erect chest film and an erect abdominal film, but if the patient is too sick to sit up, the erect films may be replaced by the left lateral decubitus view. In either case, the patient must maintain the position for a good 5 to 10 minutes, because "free air" is really not so free and actually moves slowly within the abdominal cavity. A common mistake is not to leave the patient in the erect or decubitus position long enough for air to gravitate.

Remember that both the erect views and the decubitus view should include the hemidiaphragms. Interestingly, the erect chest

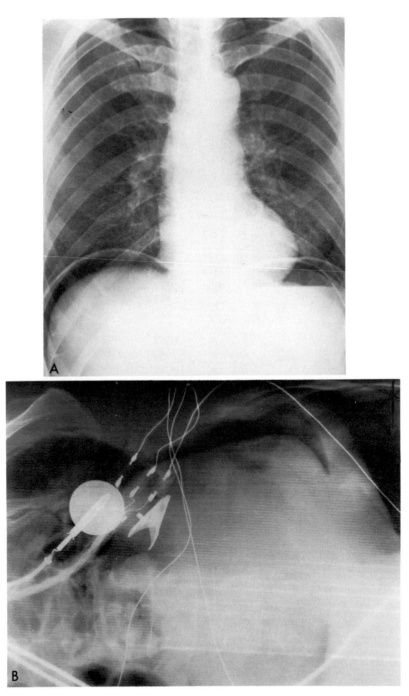

Figure 3–1. *Free air.* *A,* Erect chest x-ray, showing free air under both hemidiaphragms. The apparent appearance of two diaphragms on the left is due to a hump. *B,* Left lateral decubitus abdominal film. There is a large amount of free air over the liver. Note the sliver of air over the iliac crest. There is also an ileus pattern with scattered air fluid levels.

x-ray centered at the diaphragm is more sensitive than the erect abdominal film and will show a smaller volume of free air. Miller and Nelson (1971) were able to detect less than 1 cc of air (injected into Miller's peritoneal cavity!) on the erect chest x-ray.

All films should be correctly exposed; if the film is too light or too dark, you may make the disastrous mistake of missing free air. Making sure that films are of adequate quality is the radiologist's responsibility, and no excuses are acceptable if they are of poor quality.

Each abdominal film should be viewed in a systematic way; how the individual radiologist does this is a matter of personal preference. Eventually, it becomes an unconscious scanning procedure, but at the beginning a conscious approach is necessary. One should look for (1) abnormal gas shadows (air in or over the liver, dilatation of bowel, free or retroperitoneal air), (2) abnormal soft tissue densities (mass or ascites), and (3) abnormal calcifications. Don't forget to look at the lung bases and the bones!

The Flank Stripe

Before discussing this approach, an extremely important fat line within the abdomen, the "flank stripe," otherwise known as the properitoneal fat line (Fig. 3–2) will be described. This is the layer of fat lying immediately outside the parietal peritoneum, and as such defines the borders or limits of the peritoneal cavity. On a well-exposed abdominal film, the flank stripe will be seen to extend in a smooth curve from the rib cage to the iliac crest, where it fades out. The ascending and descending colon should be immediately medial to this fat line and separated from it by a distance of only 2 to 3 mm, the combined thickness of the peritoneum and the bowel wall itself. If the bowel is further away from the fat than a few millimeters, it has been pushed away either by a mass or by ascites.

Although the flank stripe is extremely useful in the x-ray diagnosis of ascites, it is not the earliest radiographic sign. By the time the bowel is displaced medially on x-ray, usually ascites will be detectable clinically. The first place to look for ascites is in the lesser pelvis (Fig. 3–3). Free intraperitoneal fluid will run by gravity into the lowest part of the abdomen, which means the pelvis, whether the patient is supine or erect. Fluid will collect in the cul-de-sac and the lateral recesses of the pouch of Douglas, resulting in symmetric soft tissue densities above the bladder, called "dog ears" or "Mickey Mouse" ears. This appearance is seen with only 100 to 150 ml of fluid, a degree of ascites that will not be detectable clinically. Remember, blood and ascites look the same on x-ray, so that bleeding into the peritoneum, such as occurs with a ruptured ectopic pregnancy, will look the same as a small amount of ascites. With massive ascites, the abdomen may appear very gray — the "ground-glass" appearance; if intestinal loops are gas-filled, they will float to the middle of the abdomen.

Gas Patterns on Abdominal Films

Abnormal *gas patterns* include the following:

1. Dilated but otherwise normal bowel.
2. Submucosal abnormalities, such as inflammation or ischemia, that will result in abnormal-appearing loops.
3. Signs of gangrene or potential perforation.
4. Evidence that perforation has already occurred.
5. Extraluminal gas, which suggests an abscess.

Dilated Bowel

How much bowel gas is present is extremely variable: either very little or a lot of gas may be normal. Many people are air swallowers, especially when they are sick, and a lot of bowel gas is not necessarily abnormal unless the bowel is also dilated.

Before a loop of bowel can be judged to be dilated, it must be known whether it is small bowel or colon; radiologists must therefore be able to distinguish between small and large

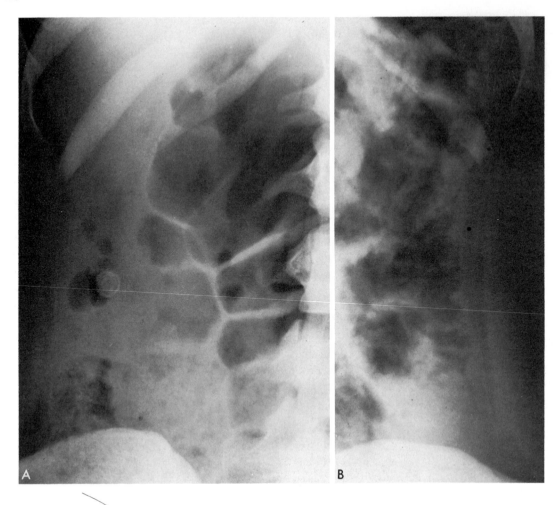

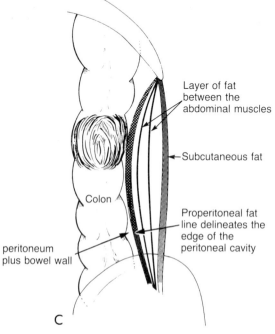

Figure 3–2. *The flank stripe. A,* Abnormal flank stripe, due to appendiceal abscess, is bulging and fuzzy in outline. Beneath the bulge there is a concentric calcification associated with what appear to be extraluminal gas collections. The lower ascending colon is closely applied to the flank stripe, but near the calcification it is displaced medially. *B, Normal flank stripe.* This extends from the lower ribs to the iliac crest and can be a thin or a thick layer of fat. The other vertical fat lines represent the fat between each layer of abdominal muscle. Note how close the descending colon is to the flank stripe. *C,* A line drawing clearly delineates the anatomy of the flank stripe.

Layer of fat between the abdominal muscles

Subcutaneous fat

Colon

Properitoneal fat line delineates the edge of the peritoneal cavity

peritoneum plus bowel wall

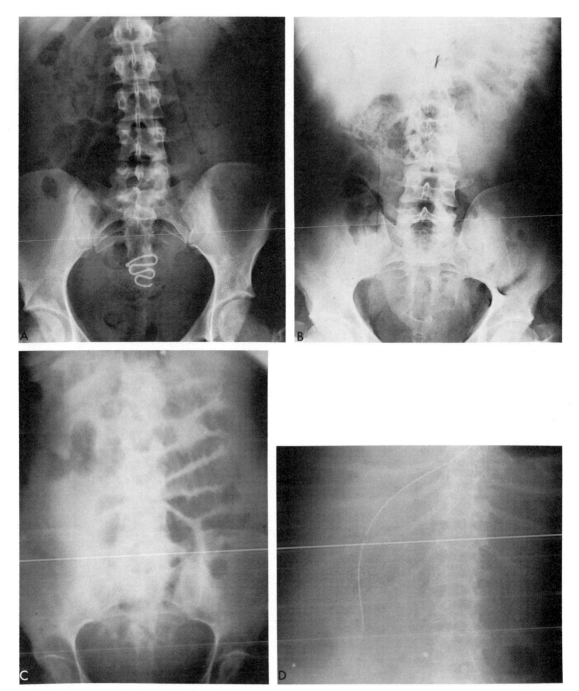

Figure 3–3. *Ascites. A,* An intrauterine device is present in the pelvis. There are bilateral symmetrical soft tissue densities on top of the bladder due to free fluid in the lateral recesses of the pouch of Douglas; this was due to hemoperitoneum from a ruptured tubal pregnancy.

B, The "Mickey Mouse" ears are evident in the pelvis. The ascending colon is markedly displaced medially from the flank stripe. Ascites was clinically evident.

C, Gas-filled loops of small bowel are displaced medially and look like they are floating on the fluid.

D, "Ground-glass" appearance. Note that there is very little gas within the abdomen and the abdomen looks gray and featureless.

bowel with a degree of certainty. Two important factors in deciding this are (1) the fold pattern within the loop, and (2) the position of that loop within the abdominal cavity.

Small bowel folds (termed "valvulae conniventes" or "plicae circulares") are fine, parallel, closely stacked soft tissue bands extending all the way across the bowel lumen. These are quite different from colonic markings (haustra), which are much further apart, are not parallel, and run only part of the way across the lumen. As for position, the colon lies peripherally, whereas the small bowel is central.

The normal diameter of small bowel loops is up to 25 to 30 mm (the size of a quarter); the criteria for the normal colon are less clearly defined. There are, however, suggested upper limits of normal above which there is an increased risk of perforation; these are a cecum greater than 9 cm across its base or a transverse colon greater than 6 cm. These measurements are only guidelines, and many patients with a colon larger than these so-called upper limits have no bowel problems; any distention must be correlated with the clinical setting. Increasing distention of the cecum is particularly ominous because there is a high risk of perforation.

The bowel will become dilated under two main circumstances: obstruction and ileus. Occasionally these may be distinguished clinically; more often the radiologist is called upon to differentiate between the two. Many times plain films alone will be diagnostic; sometimes, contrast studies, with the medium given either by mouth or by enema, are necessary to clarify.

ILEUS. An adynamic ileus will result in bowel dilatation (Fig. 3–4); without peristalsis, gas will accumulate in the paralyzed loop. Many things can cause a reflex paralytic ileus, which can be generalized or localized. Localized ileus is common near an inflammatory process, whereas generalized ileus can result from metabolic processes or drugs.

OBSTRUCTION. In obstruction, the normal passage of gas through the GI tract can no longer proceed. Air will build up proximal to the obstruction, with no air at all distally if the obstruction is complete or only a small amount

distally if it is incomplete (Fig. 3–5). Distal to the obstruction the bowel will be decompressed and smaller than usual, and proximal to the obstruction it will be dilated. This is the basis for the change in caliber seen when studying these patients with barium; the change in caliber is at the actual point of obstruction.

What might be seen in a patient with small bowel obstruction? If the obstruction is complete, there will be dilatation of small bowel and little or no gas in the colon (Fig. 3–5). In contrast, with large bowel obstruction, gas will be seen within dilated colon in a continuous column up to the obstruction, and there will be no gas distally (Fig. 3–8). There may also be secondary small bowel dilatation if the ileocecal valve (which acts as a safety valve) is incompetent. If the ileocecal valve is competent, the cecum will continue to dilate and may eventually perforate.

The question is how to proceed when obstruction is suspected? On the plain supine film, the bowel has been found to be dilated and the decision has been made in most cases whether it is small bowel or colon. The pattern may have influenced whether we think there is obstruction or ileus, although additional films may be necessary for this differentiation.

The erect film is particularly useful in this regard in small bowel obstruction. In both ileus and obstruction there is increased intraluminal gas and fluid, which result in air-fluid levels on the erect films. In obstruction, the fluid levels tend to be longer and at different heights (Figs. 3–5 to 3–7). In ileus, on the other hand, there is less fluid; the levels are shorter and at the same height.

The prone film is particularly useful in differentiating distal large bowel obstruction from colonic ileus (Fig. 3–9). If gas can be maneuvered into the rectum a high-grade obstructing lesion can be excluded. In the prone position, the rectum is the highest point within the abdomen and gas will therefore bubble up into it if the bowel is open; no gas will be seen in the rectum by this maneuver if the colon is obstructed. Naturally, it is extremely important to perform this maneuver before sigmoidoscopy and even before

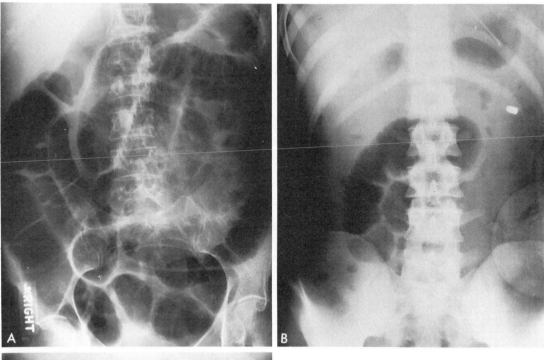

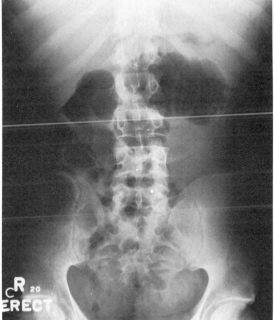

Figure 3–4. *A, Adynamic ileus.* There is generalized dilatation of both large and small bowel, affecting each equally. Gas is seen throughout the whole colon, excluding a distal obstruction. *B, Localized ileus associated with pancreatitis.* A dilated atonic-appearing loop of jejunum is present in the midabdomen. The patient had traumatic pancreatitis due to a gunshot wound (note the bullet). There is a colostomy stoma in the mid-descending colon. *C, Localized ileus and pancreatitis.* There is moderate dilatation of the transverse colon with abrupt termination just proximal to the splenic flexure; this localized ileus is known as the "colon cut-off" sign. Note the "Mickey Mouse" ears in the pelvis indicating free intraperitoneal fluid due to irritation of the peritoneum by pancreatic enzymes.

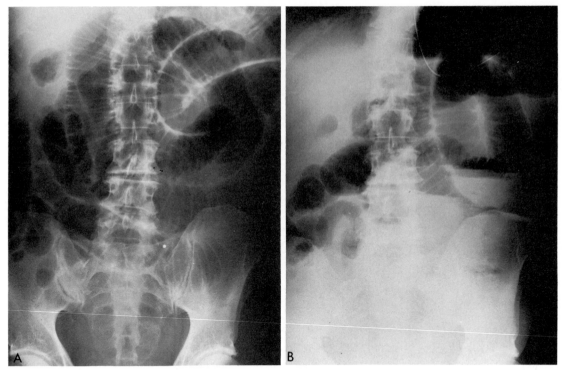

Figure 3–5. *Small bowel obstruction. A,* There is marked dilatation of small bowel extending quite distally; a small amount of gas is seen within haustra in the ascending colon. Some of the more distal loops are only faintly seen, indicating that these loops are partly fluid-filled. *B,* Multiple air-fluid levels are present, confirming the findings in *A.*

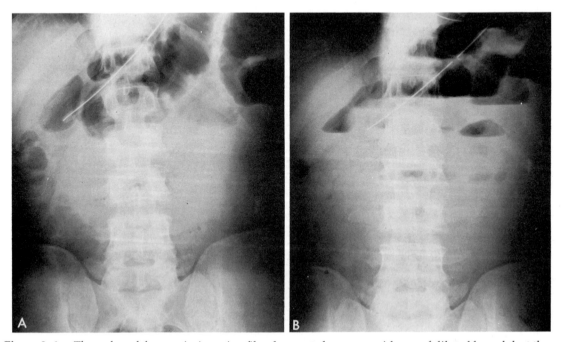

Figure 3–6. *The gasless abdomen. A,* A supine film does not show any evidence of dilated bowel, but there is mass effect in the center of the abdomen. *B,* An erect film demonstrates an unexpected finding, multiple air-fluid levels in the small bowel. There is a normal amount of colon gas. The underlying problem here was partial distal small bowel obstruction.

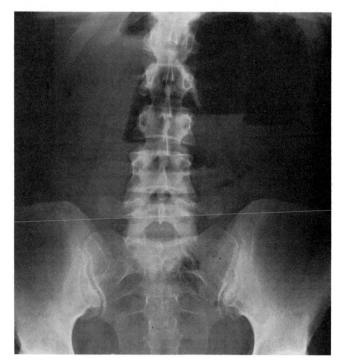

Figure 3–7. *"String of beads."* On this erect film, multiple short air-fluid levels extend in a step-ladder fashion across the left side of the abdomen. More proximally there are at least two markedly dilated loops of jejunum.

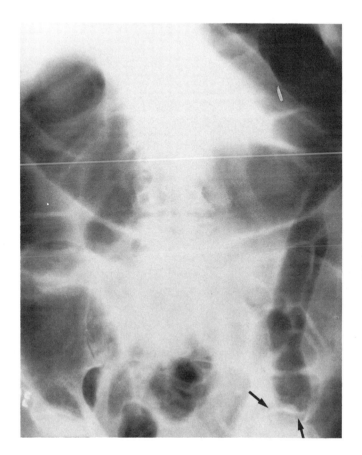

Figure 3–8. *Large bowel obstruction.* Dilated colon extends in a continuous column until the gas terminates abruptly at the junction of descending and sigmoid colon (arrows). There is no rectal air. The gas within the pelvis is within distal small bowel. The blurring is due to respiratory motion.

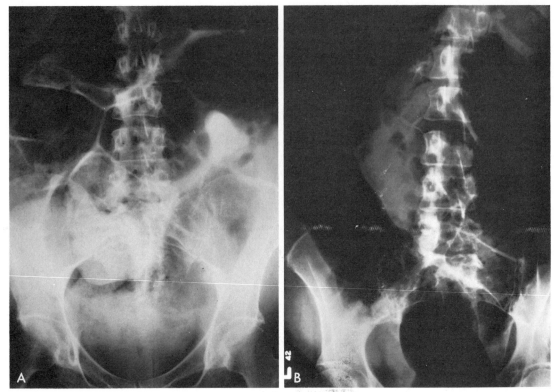

Figure 3–9. *The value of the prone film* in suspected distal colonic obstruction is well demonstrated here. *A,* Gaseous distention is present throughout the abdomen; dilated descending colon appears to stop abruptly as it enters the pelvis. *B,* By turning the patient prone, gas is now seen outlining a dilated rectum (note that the print is reproduced as if you are looking at a prone patient with the patient's left on the left).

a rectal examination, as air will be introduced through the rectum by these procedures and may give a falsely reassuring picture.

Before the contrast approach to patients with suspected bowel obstruction is discussed, other abnormal gas patterns on the plain film should be mentioned. Some of them are indications for urgent surgical intervention.

Signs of Submucosal Abnormality

Each bowel loop should be carefully scrutinized for any signs of inflammation or ischemia. These include thickened folds, thumbprinting, luminal narrowing, and separation of loops (Fig. 3–10); very late in the course, complete sloughing of the mucosa and submucosa will result in a totally featureless ap-

pearance. There is usually no peristalsis in inflamed or ischemic loops, and so they do not change in appearance from film to film.

Signs of Gangrene or Potential Perforation

PNEUMATOSIS. As already mentioned, perforation is likely to occur proximal to a large bowel obstruction. The part of the colon most at risk is the cecum, with the transverse colon running a close second. Therefore not only should the size of the colon be measured but also signs of imminent perforation should be sought. A careful search should be made for pneumatosis, the linear or mottled translucencies that indicate gas actually within the bowel wall (Fig. 3–11). As it happens, there are both "benign" and "malignant" forms of

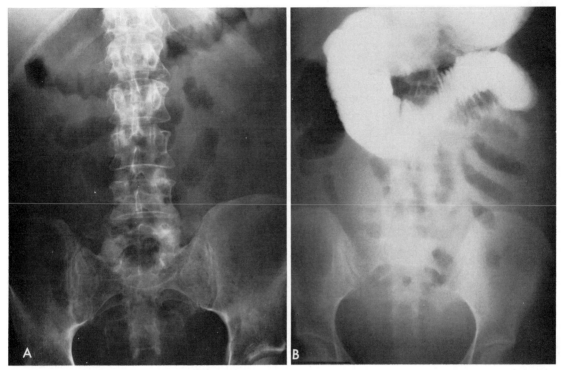

Figure 3–10. *Ischemia. A, Ischemic transverse colon.* There is thumb-printing extending along the complete length of the transverse colon. *B, Small bowel gangrene due to midgut volvulus.* Many small bowel loops are featureless, with separation of bowel loops due to wall thickening.

pneumatosis. The so-called "malignant" form indicates gangrenous bowel or bowel about to perforate from overdistention; the intramural gas has dissected in from the lumen through diseased mucosa. There is also a "benign" form (pneumatosis cystoides intestinalis), in which there are subserosal gas cysts, which also produce a mottled appearance. Benign pneumatosis is usually cystic in appearance and has been associated with many conditions, notably chronic obstructive pulmonary disease (COPD) and asthma. However, in the setting of acute abdominal symptoms, if pneumatosis is seen, it should indicate the possibility of gangrene or potential perforation; any linear or mottled translucency paralleling the wall should suggest compromised bowel. Occasionally mistakes are made, as mottling can also be seen with liquid or bloody feces. But, if mottling is seen outside the expected position of the colon, it is real cause for worry. Mottling may also indicate an abscess cavity, the gas having been released by gas-forming organisms. In addition, abscesses may result in amorphous gas collections, so that any gas collection without bowel markings within it should be suspect. Note that the mottled and amorphous appearance will not change from film to film.

GAS WITHIN LIVER. An even more ominous sign is mottled gas within the liver substance, which indicates portal pyemia. Normally on radiographs the liver is totally of soft tissue density; any gas shadows within it are abnormal and indicate gas within portal vein, biliary tree, or an abscess. Because each indicates different pathology, the radiologist must be able to differentiate among these and especially between portal vein gas and biliary tree gas. How are these two branching patterns differentiated? Recall the way bile flows and the pathway of blood in the portal vein. Bile flows toward the duodenum and thus will tend to carry gas with it out of the liver; the flow in the portal vein, on the contrary, is peripherally, toward the edge of the liver.

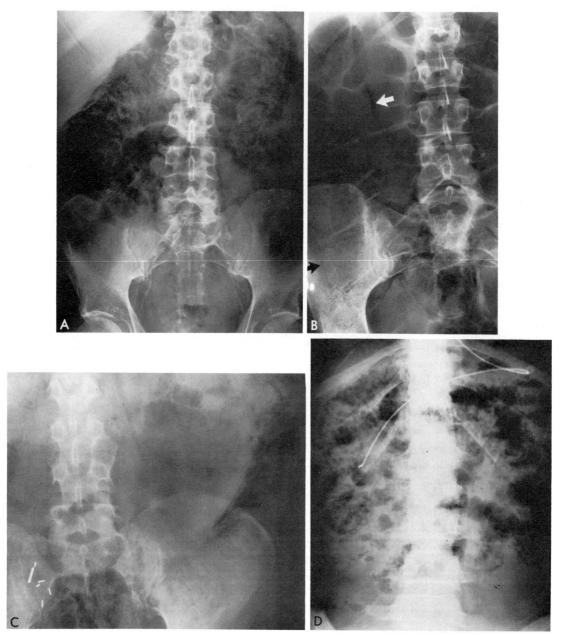

Figure 3–11. *The many manifestations of pneumatosis. A,* Multiple gas-filled collections parallel the transverse colon. This mottled appearance can be found in so-called "benign" pneumatosis, but in an acute situation it should suggest gangrene or an abscess. *B,* Linear gas (arrows) parallels the right colon in multiple areas. In the patient with an acute abdomen, this must be considered gangrene and potential perforation until proved otherwise. In this particular patient, the pneumatosis was chronic and followed a jejunoileal bypass for morbid obesity. *C,* Linear collections of gas indicate intramural dissection of air and imminent perforation. Whenever gas dissects along muscle bundles, a similar appearance can result. The patient had had a renal transplant; the incidence of both diverticulitis and sigmoid colon perforation without diverticulitis is increased in the transplant population. *D,* This appearance is due to *gangrene* of the whole small bowel. Mottled gas is seen in almost the whole of the midabdomen, occupying the space normally taken up by the small bowel.

Thus, gas in the bile ducts will be seen centrally and near the hilum; portal vein gas will be seen throughout the whole of the liver, extending almost to the periphery (Fig. 3–12). Remember, the presence of portal gas indicates an intra-abdominal catastrophe. In an adult, this finding indicates an extremely poor prognosis; in premature neonates, a condition known as necrotizing enterocolitis can result in portal vein gas, and occasionally the child survives. Biliary tree gas usually indicates a communication between the bowel and the bile ducts, either created surgically by an anastomosis or sphincterotomy, or resulting from disease, such as a fistula in gallstone ileus; occasionally infections with gas-forming organisms, such as emphysematous cholecystitis, can result in biliary tree gas.

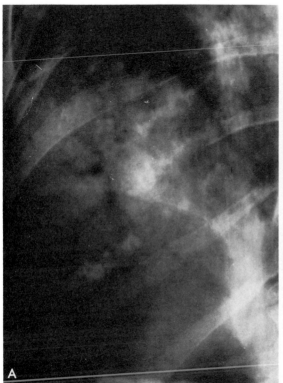
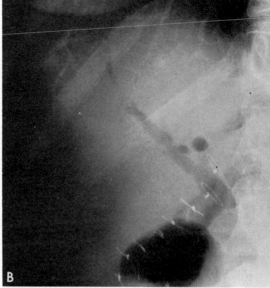
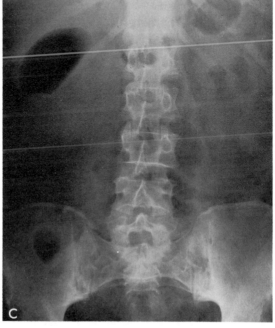

Figure 3–12. *Portal vein gas. A,* Note the mottled branching translucencies extending to the edge of the liver. *B,* Air is again visible in branching structures in the right upper quadrant. In this case, however, the air is central and at the hilum; this is the characteristic appearance of air in the biliary tree. *C, Emphysematous cholecystitis.* The oval, gas-containing structure in the right upper quadrant is the gallbladder. This patient was diabetic and developed overwhelming infection with a gas-forming organism.

Evidence of Perforation

An acute abdominal series should be performed as described previously, and a careful search made for free air under the diaphragm. Be careful not to confuse the normal subcrural fat with free air.

Occasionally gas will not be free but will remain loculated; this can happen under the edge of the liver or in the lesser sac. In the supine position, air is sometimes seen loculated over the bare area of the liver.

Even if the gas cannot be maneuvered into a position where it can be seen, there are other signs on the supine film that can provide clues that perforation has indeed already occurred. A useful sign is air on both sides of the wall, also known as the "double-wall" sign (Fig. 3–13). Here the full thickness of the bowel wall can actually be seen, instead of its width having to be inferred by visually guessing the distance between adjacent loops; the wall appears to jump out at the eyes and seems very white because air is outlining it not only from the inside but also from the outside.

Occasionally ligaments that are usually invisible will become visible if silhouetted by air. The falciform ligament may be seen in the upper abdomen or the lateral umbilical ligaments may be observed extending like an upside-down "V" in the lower abdomen.

In the "colon interposition syndrome," in which colon insinuates itself above the liver, between it and the diaphragm a false diagnosis of free air is sometimes made. Occasionally one can see haustra on the PA film in this region, but it will usually be more obvious on a lateral film.

A particularly problematical area is the assessment of gas within the abdomen following abdominal surgery. Gas remains in the peritoneal cavity following laparotomy for varying periods of time, depending on the age and body habitus of the patient. The average time it takes for gas to be resorbed is around 10 days, but more important than this is the fact that the amount of gas should continually decrease following surgery. Any increase in gas suggests perforation, perhaps of an anastomosis. An intra-abdominal drain, of course, will allow gas to be present in the abdomen for a much longer period of time without signifying trouble.

ULCER PERFORATION. If there is evidence of free air within the abdomen, the surgeon may take the patient straight to the operating room, or he may wish to know before operating exactly what has perforated. Often the clinical history will give the answer, but sometimes there are no clues. Under these circumstances a contrast study may be ordered. Most commonly perforation occurs with a peptic ulcer, usually duodenal but occasionally gastric. A limited upper GI series may be performed with *water-soluble contrast medium* (Fig. 3–15); often the patient is too sick for a complete upper GI series to be performed, but most perforated ulcers can be demonstrated by giving contrast medium by mouth and then placing the patient on his right side. A film taken some 10 minutes later may show the perforation unless the leaking ulcer is on the anterior wall; then the leak may not be demonstrated unless the patient is turned onto his stomach.

COLONIC PERFORATION. The clinician may suspect that it is the colon that has perforated; this could be due to a perforated diverticulum, a perforated cancer, or perforation of a normal colon proximal to a distal obstruction. Remember that although diverticulitis may result in free air, more often surrounding inflammation will result in the perforation being sealed off to form an abscess.

If the colon has perforated, performing a contrast study from below will result in even more stool being pushed out into the general peritoneal cavity. Experimentally, any enema in this situation, even a saline enema, increases the morbidity and mortality. Many would advise, therefore, that no contrast enema be performed if there is free air. It is safer to give water-soluble contrast by mouth, demonstrate that the upper GI tract is intact, and, by exclusion, make the presumption that the lower tract is the culprit.

RETROPERITONEAL PERFORATION. Perforation of a *retroperitoneal* structure will not result in free air within the peritoneal cavity, but will produce retroperitoneal air. The duodenum, except for the bulb, is retroperitoneal, as is part of the sigmoid and the ascending

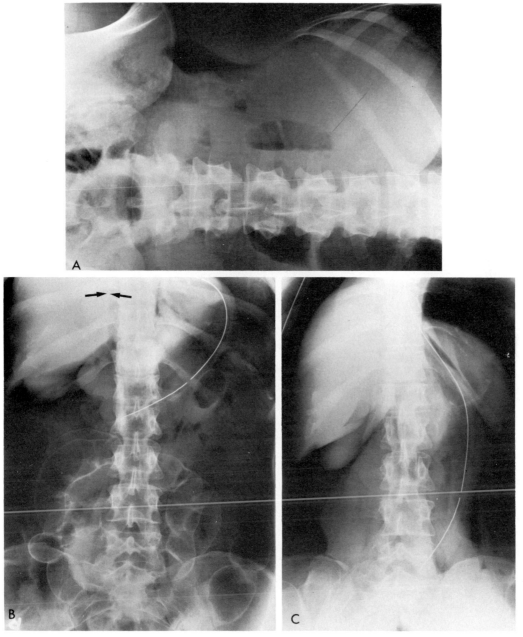

Figure 3–13. *Other manifestations of free air. A, Air over the iliac crest.* In this decubitus film note that there is an amorphous collection of air over the iliac crest; there is no evidence of free air in the usual position over the liver. This was indeed free air and moved when the patient was brought upright.

B, The "double-wall sign." Air is seen outlining the lateral and inferior borders of the liver and the gallbladder. The "double-wall sign" is clearly evident due to both intra- and extraluminal air. Air has dissected up under the left crus. The falciform ligament (arrows) is clearly seen.

C, "Free air" from a diagnostic pneumoperitoneum. The liver and spleen are clearly outlined, as is the left crus of the diaphragm and the gallbladder. A nasogastric tube is in the stomach.

Illustration continued on following page.

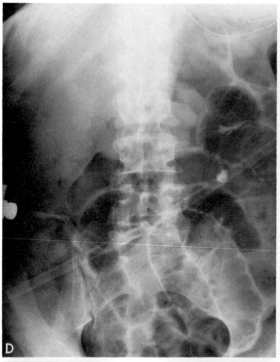

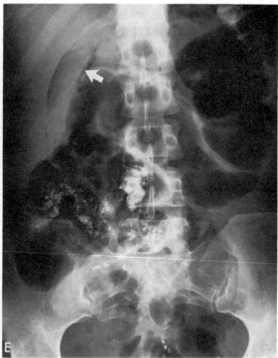

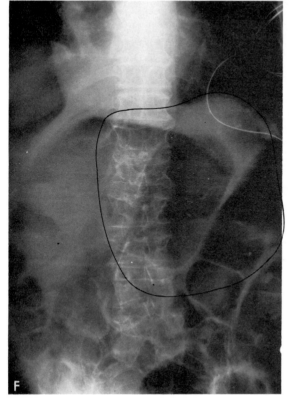

Figure 3–13 *Continued*

D, Right upper quadrant features. The right upper quadrant often offers important clues to the presence of perforation. The falciform ligament is clearly outlined. A relative area of lucency is seen over the liver. Incidentally, calcified gallstones are present. There is a generalized ileus.

E, Air is seen outlining the kidney in Morison's pouch and trapped under the edge of the liver (arrow). A generalized ileus pattern is present, and residual barium is seen from a previous contrast study.

F, Pneumoperitoneum: air in the lesser sac? There is a large amorphous gas collection in the upper abdomen suggesting extraluminal air. The expected position of air in the lesser sac is drawn on the film and superimposed upon this gas collection. To determine whether the extraluminal air is in the lesser sac or trapped under the anterior abdominal wall, a cross-table lateral film would be helpful.

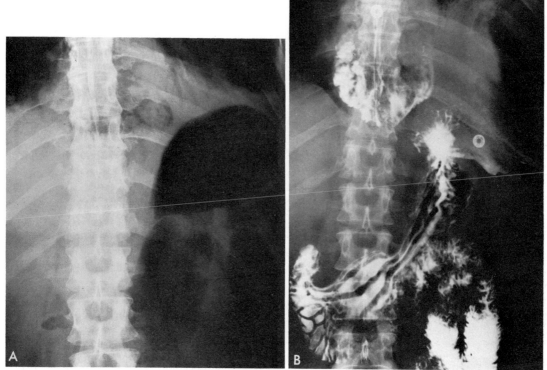

Figure 3–14. *Boerhaave's syndrome* (spontaneous perforation of the esophagus). *A,* Plain film of the abdomen and lower thorax demonstrates what appears to be extraluminal gas. This is gas in the mediastinum as it crosses the midline and therefore cannot be intraparenchymal (in lung). An air bronchogram is seen in the retrocardiac area and the left hemidiaphragm is obscured. The appearances are those of perforation/abscess in the mediastinum with an associated pneumonic process. *B,* Proceeding to contrast examination, extravasation of contrast material into both the mediastinum and the abdominal cavity, where it is tracking along the under surface of the spleen, is seen. The esophageal tear was straddling the left hemidiaphragm.

and descending colon. Characteristically, retroperitoneal air will dissect up and down the muscle bundles of the psoas and will result in streaky translucencies (Fig. 3–16). Remember, the iliopsoas muscle continues down into the thigh, and gas can dissect out of the abdomen into the leg. There have even been cases of ruptured diverticula that have presented as crepitus in the ankle!

ABSCESS. The radiologist should also make a careful search for any extraluminal gas, which would suggest an abscess. Again the search is for either a mottled gas collection that is not in the expected location of the bowel or

an amorphous collection of gas lacking bowel markings (Fig. 3–17). This appearance will not change from film to film as abscesses are contained loculations. If an intra-abdominal abscess is suspected, often the plain film will not show any abnormality, and it will be necessary to perform ultrasound or computed tomography to make the diagnosis of an abscess.

Basically, then, one has to decide what the underlying process is and whether there are any danger signs. Can a complete diagnosis be made on plain films alone, or must contrast studies be done? Which contrast

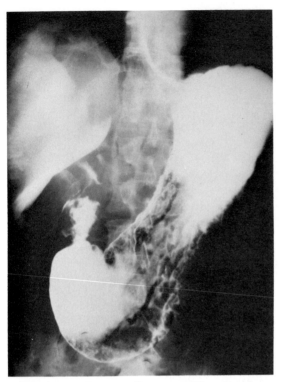

Figure 3–15. Gastrografin upper GI series shows extravasation of contrast medium from the region of the duodenal bulb, although an actual ulcer crater has not been demonstrated. Contrast medium is pooling up under the edge of the liver.

study is indicated, i.e., barium versus water-soluble contrast? Should this medium be given orally or by enema?

Some common clinical situations will now be considered.

Does the Patient Have Obstruction?

If dilated loops of bowel are seen, first try to decide whether they represent ileus or obstruction; sometimes this is easy, but more frequently it is difficult. If obstruction is suspected, it is necessary to identify whether the small bowel or the colon is involved because the way contrast medium is used to make the diagnosis differs depending on which part of the bowel is involved.

Another important question is whether the obstruction is partial or complete. A partial small bowel obstruction may resolve itself,

whereas a complete obstruction requires urgent surgery; large bowel obstruction, whether partial or complete, rarely resolves by itself.

SMALL BOWEL OBSTRUCTION. As already mentioned, a complete obstruction can be diagnosed on plain abdominal films alone by seeing dilated small bowel, no gas in the colon, and air-fluid levels of the erect film. Often, however, the picture is not as classic as this, and a contrast study is necessary for clarification. The questions in this case are whether to give barium, how to give it, and whether barium by mouth is dangerous in suspected cases of small bowel obstruction (Table 3–1).

This last question has caused many a problem. Barium by mouth is safe in small bowel obstruction, as the preparation will remain liquid and will not become impacted or turn to "concrete" as many surgeons fear; this is because in the small bowel above the obstruction there is a large volume of in-

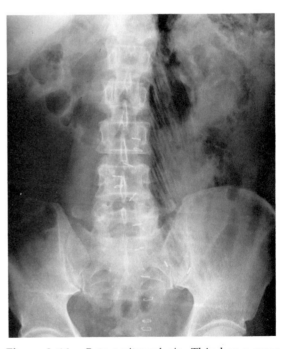

Figure 3–16. *Retroperitoneal air.* This has a very distinctive appearance. As the air dissects along the muscle bundles of the retroperitoneum, a streaky appearance results. In this particular patient, a retroperitoneal anastomosis had ruptured one week following surgery.

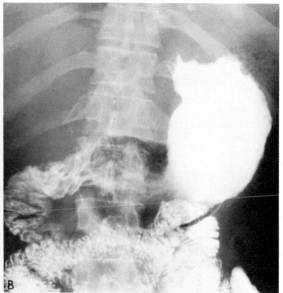

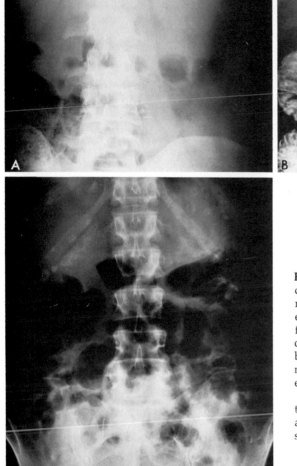

Figure 3–17. *Abscess* (subphrenic) *A,* A mottled collection of gas in the left upper quadrant (arrow) raises the question of an abscess. Note the markedly increased distance between the gastric fundus and the diaphragm, indicating a space-occupying lesion. *B,* The patient has been given barium to outline the fundus of the stomach; the mottled gas in the left upper quadrant is indeed extragastric.

C, Pelvic abscess. There is a soft tissue mass in the pelvis; multiple extraluminal gas collections are within the mass. This was a diverticular abscess.

traluminal fluid. *In colonic obstruction, however, barium by mouth is contraindicated.* The colon above the obstruction will perform its normal function and will resorb water from the barium, resulting in concrete. If, therefore, there is any doubt on the plain films whether the suspected obstruction is in the small bowel or the colon (and this will happen in a surprising number of cases) (Fig. 3–18), it is much safer to do a barium enema first. After having proved the colon normal, the small bowel obstruction can be tackled in two ways: either the barium enema can be continued and an attempt made to reflux barium through the

TABLE 3–1. CHOICE OF CONTRAST MEDIUM

	Indications	Contraindications
BARIUM	To demonstrate *anatomy* and *mucosal detail* anywhere in the GI tract	Known or suspected *perforation*
	In partial small bowel obstruction — to show *site* and *cause*	Should not be given from above in suspected *large bowel obstruction*
GASTROGRAFIN	Known or suspected *perforation* ? Complete small bowel obstruction ? Ileus versus obstruction ? Diverticulitis	Known or suspected *aspiration* Suspected communication with the lung

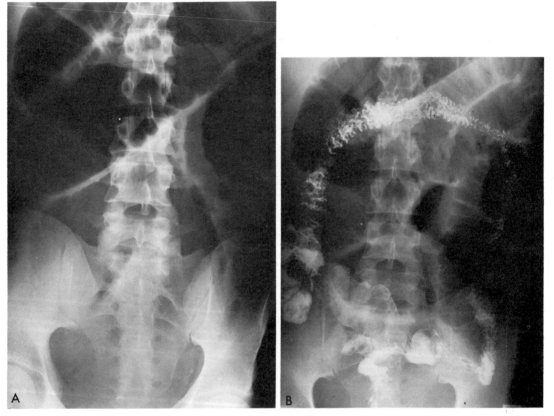

Figure 3–18. *Small bowel obstruction simulating large bowel obstruction.*

A, There is massive dilatation of bowel in the upper abdomen, and it is extremely diffcult to decide whether this is small bowel or colon. Most people would say it was dilated colon. In fact, this was massively dilated distal small bowel resulting from obstruction at the ileocecal valve. Note that no gas is seen in the rectum, nor in the right iliac fossa or descending colon region.

B, A barium enema was performed, which showed a normal colon. It was possible to reflux a small amount of barium into the terminal ileum proximal to the obstructing lesion, which was in the last 1 cm of the small bowel. At surgery, Crohn's disease was found.

ileocecal valve, thus reaching the obstruction from below, or a small bowel follow-through can be done with barium from above (Fig. 3–19). In cases of *distal* small bowel obstruction, a retrograde small bowel enema is often the fastest way to make the diagnosis of the site and cause of the obstruction: a barium study from above is a much slower process,

and it may take many hours for the barium to reach the level of obstruction.

Films are taken at intervals determined by how fast the barium is progressing, the aim being to find the site and cause of the obstruction. In complete obstruction, the barium column will terminate abruptly; in partial obstruction there is a sudden change in caliber

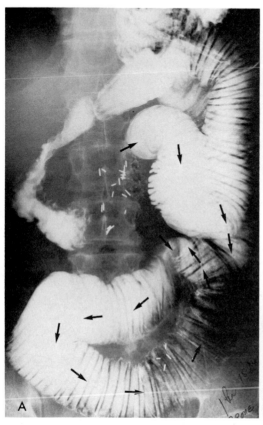

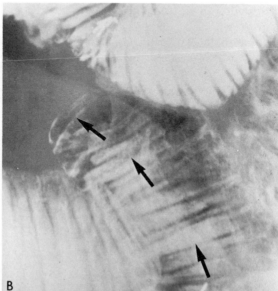

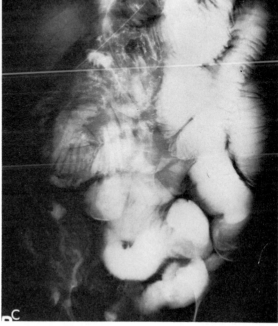

Figure 3–19. *Small bowel obstruction due to adhesions.*

A, On small bowel follow-through, marked dilatation of the small bowel with normal valvulae conniventes is seen. There is complete obstruction to the flow of barium in the mid–small bowel.

B, A close-up film shows a sharp vertical cut-off, which is the classic appearance of an adhesion.

C, *Partial small bowel obstruction* (with oral barium). There is dilatation of small bowel down to the pelvis, where there is a sudden change in caliber from dilated to decompressed (smaller than normal) small bowel. The actual obstructing point would be found by fluoroscopy; in this particular patient, obstruction was due to an adhesion.

between dilated preobstruction and decompressed postobstruction bowel (Fig. 3–19). Having found the site, fluoroscopy may be needed to define the cause. The most common cause of small bowel obstruction is adhesions, but other diseases, such as Crohn's disease, lymphoma, or metastases, may present in this way.

A little digression about the use of Gastrografin in cases of suspected small bowel obstruction is in order. There is *no* justification for use of oral Gastrografin to define the site and cause of a partial small bowel obstruction. Gastrografin will become extremely diluted in this clinical situation, owing both to its own extreme hyperosmolality (7 to 10 times the osmolarity of plasma) and to the large amount of intraluminal fluid which is an accompaniment of small bowel obstruction. Because of the hyperosmolar effect, Gastrografin may even be harmful in a patient with borderline dehydration, because it draws fluid from the blood.

Some have advocated the use of a small amount of Gastrografin orally to differentiate complete small bowel obstruction (requiring urgent surgery) from incomplete obstruction (when presumably urgent surgery is not necessary). When this is done, identifying Gastrografin in the colon excludes a complete obstruction.

COLONIC OBSTRUCTION. It may occasionally be difficult to differentiate between distal large bowel obstruction and an ileus. The value of a prone film in many of these cases has already been discussed and the findings on the prone film may obviate the need for a contrast study. Even if the patient definitely has obstruction as seen on the plain films, the surgeon may still wish to know what is causing the obstruction. The most common causes of colonic obstruction in Western society are carcinoma (Fig. 3–21) and diverticuli-

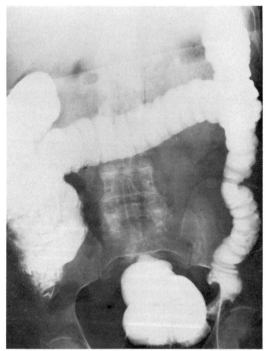

Figure 3–21. *Sigmoid colon carcinoma.* Barium enema demonstrates an applecore lesion at the junction of the descending and sigmoid colon. In the presence of high-grade obstruction, it is a mistake to let such a large amount of contrast medium flow proximal to the obstructing lesion. The aim is merely to show what is causing the obstruction and how extensive the lesion is.

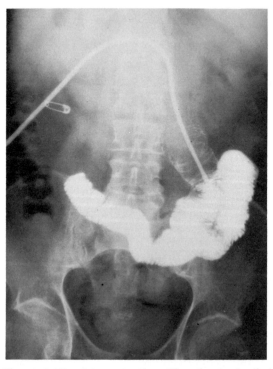

Figure 3–20. *Intussusception.* The classic "coiled spring" appearance is illustrated; the appearance results from barium trying to squeeze past the intussusception.

tis, with volvulus accounting for only some 10 per cent of cases.

If a contrast study is performed, it should be limited to showing the level and cause of the obstruction. In the acute situation, the radiologist is not trying to examine the whole colon; the extent is merely to dribble enough barium past the obstructing lesion to define it adequately. It is most important not to allow a large volume of barium to flow through the obstructing lesion. This would be tantamount to giving barium by mouth: the result is a concrete mess. To this end, barium is run in very slowly under careful fluoroscopic monitoring. Remember, once barium appears in *dilated* colon, presumably it has already passed the obstruction; do not run in any more barium but try to find the obstructing lesion by unwinding the colon. If there is complete obstruction to retrograde flow of contrast medium, giving glucagon may help by relieving any associated spasm.

VOLVULUS. A less common cause of large bowel obstruction in Western society is *volvulus*. A quite different situation exists in some other countries, such as Iran, Finland, and Russia, where up to 90 per cent of large bowel obstruction is due to volvulus. The basic anatomy necessary for volvulus is a very long mesentery with a very short attachment of its base. This most commonly occurs in the sigmoid colon and the cecum.

Sigmoid Volvulus (Fig. 3–22). The sigmoid colon dilates and twists on its base, resulting in a closed loop obstruction; proximal to the twist the large bowel will dilate. The twisted loop itself forms a configuration known as an upside-down "U." If the abdomen seems to be overfilled with dilated colon, sigmoid volvulus should also be strongly considered.

Cecal Volvulus. With volvulus of the cecum, on the other hand, the cecum twists out of the right iliac fossa and into the center of the abdomen (Fig. 3–23); in such cases there

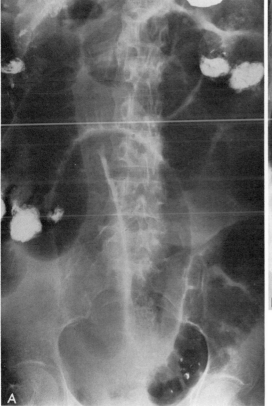
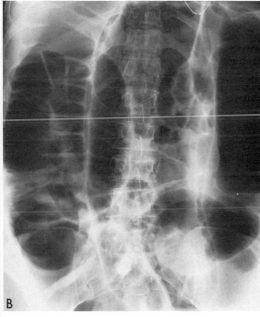

Figure 3–22. *Sigmoid volvulus. A,* There is an unusual gas collection in the midabdomen with an upside-down "U" configuration; the thick white line in the center of this points to the site of the twist. *B,* A more massive dilatation can take place, as is demonstrated in this film.

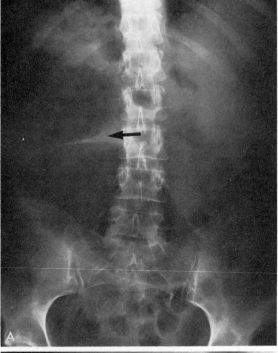

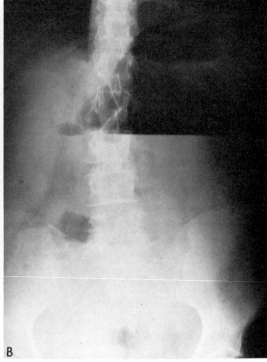

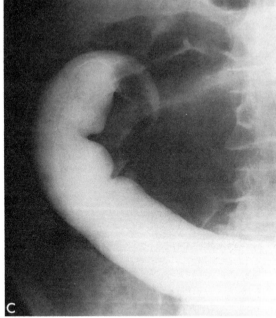

Figure 3–23. *Cecal volvulus.*

A, There is an unusual, amorphous, gas-containing collection in the right midabdomen. No other abnormal loops of bowel are seen. With some imagination, the ileocecal valve (arrow) can be defined; note that the cecum cannot be identified in the right lower quadrant.

B, An erect film reveals double air-fluid levels in the left upper quadrant — the "double stomach" sign. This is due to an air-fluid level in the stomach and in the cecum.

C, On barium enema, there is the classic appearance of volvulus, the "beaking" or "bird-of-prey" outline to the advancing edge of barium.

is a large gas collection in the midabdomen, no identifiable colon gas, and a distal small bowel obstruction. An erect film in cecal volvulus will demonstrate the so-called "double stomach" sign, with air-fluid levels both in the stomach and in the cecum. (This should not be confused with the "double bubble" sign of duodenal atresia, in which the air-fluid levels are on different sides of the spine.)

Many times these diagnoses can be made on plain films, but often contrast studies are necessary. With contrast there is a classic appearance to the leading edge of the barium, the "beaking" or "bird-of-prey" appearance, caused by the barium trying to force its way through the twist. Occasionally in cases of sigmoid volvulus — and many of these cases are anecdotal — a barium enema may not only be diagnostic but therapeutic as well. Occasionally the volvulus may reduce during the enema, and gentle attempts at such reduction should be made. Attempts at reduction should be limited to volvulus of the sigmoid colon; attempting to reduce cecal volvulus by barium enema is not advised.

Remember, as with any closed loop obstruction, the chance that a strangulated loop is present is high; early diagnosis is therefore essential (Fig. 3–24).

Does the Patient Have Diverticulitis?

This is one of the most common questions the radiologist will be asked. If the patient has fever, left lower quadrant pain, tenderness, and an abdominal mass, a clinical diagnosis of acute diverticulitis can be made; x-ray studies are not necessary in these cases. Indeed, a barium enema in this "hot" patient could even be dangerous and result in perforation or gram-negative septicemia. In some patients, however, acute diverticulitis is the provisional diagnosis, but the clinical findings are less specific. It is in these patients that radiology may be helpful and a barium enema may be requested.

How the study is done is very important.

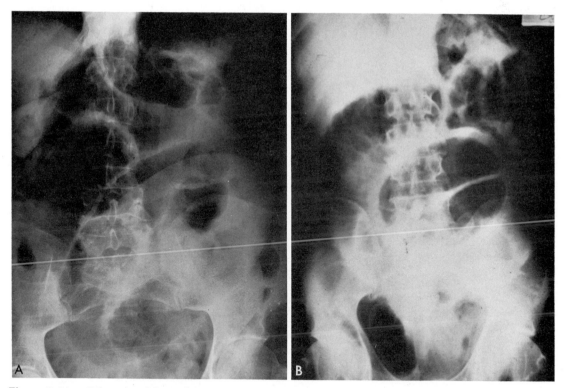

Figure 3–24. *Other closed loop obstructions;* pseudotumor and coffee-bean signs. *A,* A football-shaped mass is seen in the left midabdomen, and proximal to this the small bowel is markedly dilated. Note, in the right lower quadrant, how faintly visible the valvulae are, indicating partly fluid-filled loops. An opacified gallbladder is seen in the right upper quadrant. The presence of a large amount of fluid within the closed loop suggests strangulating obstruction. The pseudotumor is simply a coffee-bean–shaped structure containing fluid instead of air. *B,* A gas-containing loop with the appearance of a coffee-bean on its side is seen in the midabdomen. If this were turned 90 degrees or in the pelvis, it would look exactly like sigmoid volvulus.

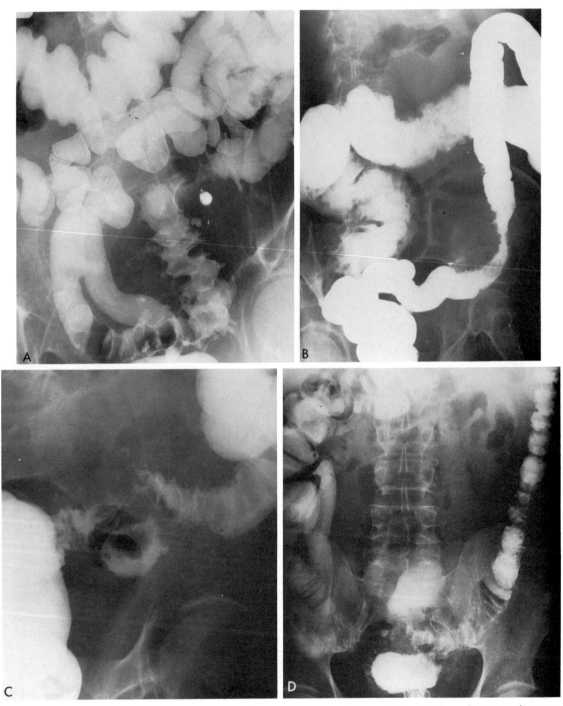

Figure 3–25 *See legend on opposite page*

The barium (or Gastrografin) should be run in slowly under low pressure (keep the enema bag low), watching carefully for mass effect or extravasation. The moment either of these findings is encountered, terminate the study. A study limited to the sigmoid colon is adequate in most cases.

Which contrast medium is chosen is personal preference. Although expensive, Gastrografin may be preferable, as extravasation may occur. Another reason for using Gastrografin is its rapid absorption; this overcomes the problem of extravasated contrast medium remaining in the diseased area, which could confuse follow-up studies.

There are stringent criteria for making the x-ray diagnosis of acute diverticulitis (Fig. 3–25). The presence of diverticula, muscular hypertrophy, and spasm is not enough, as these are part and parcel of diverticulosis. Recall the pathology of diverticulitis: the basic fact is microperforation of a diverticulum, resulting in peridiverticulitis and an abscess; surrounding inflammation may result in a fistula. So, on x-ray, extravasation into a cavity, or a fistula, or an extrinsic mass effect due to the abscess will be seen; there may be associated serosal inflammation (spiculation and tethering). A postevacuation film is ex-

tremely important; it may show more extensive extravasation. Glucagon may also be extremely useful, since it relieves associated spasm. Diverticulitis should be especially borne in mind in certain high-incidence groups, such as renal transplant and dialysis patients. It is particularly important to make the diagnosis in these patients, as signs and symptoms of disease may be masked by steroid and immunosuppressive medication. Radiology may first uncover this complication and thus allow early treatment.

Does the Patient Have Appendicitis?

Certainly this question is not meant to imply that appendicitis should be diagnosed by x-ray. Usually this diagnosis is made on clinical grounds, and even plain films are not requested. If a plain film is taken in suspected cases, it may be completely normal. In approximately 10 per cent of patients with appendicitis, a calcification may be seen in the right lower quadrant, the appendicolith. Other signs include a localized small bowel ileus in the right lower quadrant, a few short air-fluid levels on the upright film, or a soft tissue mass.

Figure 3–25. *Diverticulitis. A, Mass effect.* A full-column enema shows sigmoid diverticulosis and muscular hypertrophy. On the inferior aspect of the colon, at the junction of the descending and sigmoid, there is an extrinsic mass effect consistent with pressure from an abscess cavity. Barium from a previous barium enema has remained in the diverticulum. Barium obstructing the neck of a diverticulum theoretically could result in diverticulitis and has been implicated in some cases by several authors.

B, A Gastrografin enema reveals an abnormality at the junction of the descending colon and sigmoid colon. There is narrowing of the lumen associated with spiculation and mass effect and some extravasation of contrast medium distally. Multiple mottled gas collections are seen within the bowel wall, indicating a pericolic abscess.

C, In the sigmoid colon, in addition to luminal narrowing, spiculation, and angulation, there is extravasation of Gastrografin into a cavity (abscess cavity). Although no diverticula are seen, the surrounding spasm and inflammatory changes indicate an inflammatory etiology.

D, The postevacuation film from the same patient shows even more extravasation. This often happens following active contraction of the colon; sometimes the postevacuation film is the *only* film to show extravasation and it is a *vital* film if this diagnosis is suspected.

Occasionally the radiologist is asked to perform a barium enema to exclude this diagnosis. A full barium enema in these cases is not necessary and since most of the patients are very young, a limited study concentrating on the cecal area is advised. The aim is to fill the appendix completely. It has been found that with good colonic distention, and both a postevacuation film and a follow-up film 2 hours following the study, the appendix can be filled in 85 per cent of people. Whether glucagon helps to fill the appendix or not is unknown. If the appendix can be filled completely to its bulbous end, appendicitis can be excluded. Nonfilling of the appendix in the appropriate clinical situation is presumptive evidence of disease; complete filling excludes the diagnosis, incomplete filling is nonspecific.

Other signs indicating a mass in the right lower quadrant are sometimes seen, such as extrinsic defects or inflammatory changes on the cecum, both of which indicate a periappendiceal abscess.

Although these findings may be helpful in selected patients, we must reiterate that in most cases of acute appendicitis, the diagnosis is made clinically, without resorting to radiologic procedures.

Portable Studies of the GI Tract

The question could be asked: Are these of any value at all or are they completely useless?

Occasionally, when performing a small bowel follow-through, the patient is so ill that it would be dangerous to keep him in the x-ray department for the time necessary to complete the small bowel evaluation. Under these circumstances, having administered the contrast medium under fluoroscopy, follow-up portable films may be performed, and these may define the level of the obstruction. Fluoroscopy, however, is extremely important to pinpoint the exact site and cause of the obstruction.

There is, however, *absolutely no place for a portable study of the colon*. There are many risks attendant upon an emergency barium enema, the gravest of which is colonic perforation. Fluoroscopy is essential to watch for overdistention, to see that the barium (or Gastrografin) is running well, and, even more important, to look for contrast extravasation. All contrast studies of the colon should therefore be performed under fluoroscopic control.

The Patient with an Acute Upper or Lower GI Bleed

In this section the patient with hematemesis, hematochezia, melena, or a sudden drop in hematocrit will be discussed. Under these clinical circumstances, a number of decisions have to be made before proceeding with any contrast study.

First to be determined is whether the patient is bleeding acutely at present and, if so, how fast. If the patient is bleeding profusely, angiography is the procedure of choice, both to find the source of the blood loss and to institute therapy to control the hemorrhage. If, however, the patient is bleeding at a slower rate (less than 2 ml per minute), angiography usually will not show the bleeding site. Under these circumstances the question is whether to choose a contrast study or endoscopy. With acute bleeding, the yield of both studies is much lower than in the chronic situation; blood or clots within the lumen interfere both with direct vision and with coating. If endoscopy is being considered, however, this should be performed before any barium is introduced into the bowel. In lower GI bleeding, a barium enema in an unprepared patient is unlikely to be fruitful in the search for bleeding polyps. Only gross lesions, such as a large constricting lesion, ischemic colitis, or diverticulosis, may be found. If emergency studies are negative, a repeat examination following adequate preparation will be necessary to look for other sources of bleeding.

Abdominal Trauma

Under this heading will be discussed not the patient with trauma to the liver, spleen, or kidneys but trauma to the GI tract itself. Certain parts of the bowel, being fixed in relation to the spine, are particularly susceptible to blunt abdominal trauma. The small bowel and those parts of the colon on a mesentery will move out of the way of a glancing blow; the fixed C-sweep, pancreas, and retroperitoneal tissues cannot move. Damage to the retroperitoneal duodenum produces an intramural hematoma and may even result in retroperitoneal perforation. If a hematoma forms, it will usually resolve by itself, but occasionally it becomes so huge that duodenal obstruction occurs and surgical evacuation is necessary. The radiologist may be asked to perform a Gastrografin study of the duodenal C-sweep to exclude a duodenal rupture or an intramural hemorrhage.

Similarly, blunt trauma may result in traumatic pancreatitis, and the findings here are similar to those of pancreatitis from any other cause.

Retroperitoneal hemorrhage is extremely difficult to diagnose on plain films, although occasionally loss of a psoas outline (a very unreliable sign) or generalized ileus may suggest the diagnosis. Contrast studies are not indicated, and computed tomography is probably the procedure of choice (although ultrasound may be helpful) in suspected cases of retroperitoneal hemorrhage.

References

General

The acute abdomen. Part I. Bowel obstruction. Semin Roentgenol 8:281–338, 1973.
The acute abdomen. Part II. Inflammatory disease. Semin Roentgenol 8:365–464, 1973.
Dietz MW: Lesser peritoneal sac abnormalities. Mo. Med. 66:106–109, 1969.
Frimann-Dahl J: Roentgen Examinations in Acute Abdominal Diseases. Springfield, Ill., Charles C Thomas, 1974.
Mellins HZ (Ed): Radiologic diagnosis of acute abdominal disease. Radiol Clin North Am 2:1–183, 1964.
Menuck L, Siemers PT: Pneumoperitoneum: Importance of right upper quadrant features. Am J Roentgenol 127:753–756, 1976.
Meyers MA: Colonic ileus. Gastrointest Radiol 2:37–40, 1977.
Meyers MA, Oliphant M: Pitfalls and pickups in plain-film diagnosis of the abdomen. Curr Probl Radiol 4:3–27, 1974.
Moss AA, Goldberg HI, Brotman M: Idiopathic intestinal pseudo-obstruction. Am J Roentgenol 115:312, 1972.
Nelson SW: Extraluminal gas collections due to diseases of the gastrointestinal tract. Am J Roentgenol 115:225–248, 1972.
Schuffler MD, Rohrmann CA Jr, Templeton FE: The radiologic manifestations of idiopathic intestinal pseudoobstruction. Am J Roentgenol 127:729, 1976.
Walker LA, Weens HS: Radiological observations of the lesser peritoneal sac. Radiology 80:727, 1963.
Whalen JP, Berne AS II: Roentgen interpretation of pathologic alterations. Radiology 92:473–480, 1969.
Whalen JP, Berne AS, Riemenschneider PA: The extraperitoneal periviscereal fat pad. I. Its role in the roentgenologic visualization of abdominal organs. Radiology 92:466–472, 1969.

Technical

Laufer I: The left lateral view in the plain-film assessment of abdominal distention. Radiology 119:265–269, 1976.
Miller RE: The technical approach to the acute abdomen. Semin Roentgenol 8:267–279, 1973.
Miller RE, Nelson SW: The roentgenologic demonstration of tiny amounts of free intraperitoneal gas: experimental and clinical studies. Am J Roentgenol 112:574–585, 1971.

Pneumatosis

Bloch C: The natural history of pneumatosis coli. Radiology 123:311–314, 1977.
Olmsted WW, Madewell JE: Pneumatosis cystoides intestinalis: A pathophysiologic explanation of the roentgenographic signs. Gastrointest Radiol 1:177–181, 1976.
Marshak RH, Lindner AE, Maklansky D: Pneumatosis cystoides coli. Gastrointest Radiol 2:85–89, 1977.
Meyers MA, Ghahremani GG, Clements JL Jr, Goodman K: Pneumatosis intestinalis. Gastrointest Radiol 2:91–105, 1977.

Abscess

Halber MD, Daffner RH, Morgan CL, Trought WS, Thompson WM, Rice RP, Korobkin M: Intraabdominal abscess: Current concepts in radiologic evaluation. Am J Roentgenol 133:9, 1979.
Whalen JP: Anatomy and radiologic diagnosis of perihepatic abscesses. Symposium on the alimentary tract. Radiol Clin North Am 14:406, 1976.

Volvulus

Abrams HL, Waas WA: The diagnosis of volvulus of the cecum. Radiology 60:36–45, 1953.
Figiel LS, Figiel SJ: Sigmoid volvulus. Variations in the roentgen pattern. Am J Roentgenol 81:683–693, 1959.
Kerry RL, Lee F, Ransom HK: Roentgenologic examination in the diagnosis and treatment of colon volvulus. Am J Roentgenol 113:343–348, 1971.
Ritvo M, Golden JL: The roentgen diagnosis of volvulus of the sigmoid with intestinal obstruction. Am J Roentgenol 56:480–488, 1946.

Diverticulitis

Homer MJ, Danford RO: Acute diverticulitis in the young adult. Radiology 125:623–626, 1977.
Julien PJ, Goldberg HI, Margulis AR, Belzer FO: Gastrointestinal complications following renal transplantation. Radiology 117:37–43, 1975.
Meyers MA, Alonso DR, Baer JW: Pathogenesis of massively bleeding colonic diverticulosis: New obstructions. Am J Roentgenol 127:901–908, 1976.
Wolf BS, Khilnani M, Marshak RH: Diverticulosis and diverticulitis: Roentgen findings and their interpretation. Am J Roentgenol 77:726–743, 1957.

Appendicitis

Balthazar EJ, Gade M: The normal and abnormal development of the appendix. A radiographic assessment. Radiology 121:599–604, 1976.
Homer MJ, Braver JM: Recurrent appendicitis: Reexamination of a controversial disease. Gastrointest Radiol 4:295–302, 1979.
Sakover RP, Del Fava RL: Frequency of visualization of the normal appendix with the barium enema examination. Am J Roentgenol 121:312–317, 1974.
Vaudagna JS, McCort JJ: Plain film diagnosis of retrocecal appendicitis. Radiology 117:533–536, 1975.

Bleeding

Athanasoulis CA, Waltman AC, Novelline RA, Krudy AG, Sniderman KW: Angiography: Its contribution to the emergency management of gastrointestinal hemorrhage. Radiol Clin North Am 14:265–280, 1976.
Briley CA Jr, Jackson DC, Johnsrude IS, Mills SR: Acute gastrointestinal hemorrhage of small-bowel origin. Radiology 136:317–319, 1980.
Han SY, Witten DM, Prim HS: Plain film findings in massive gastrointestinal bleeding. Am J Roentgenol 128:437–440, 1977.
Higgins CB, Bookstein JJ, Davis GB, Galloway DC, Barr JW: Therapeutic embolization for intractable chronic bleeding. Radiology 122:473–478, 1977.
Johnsrude IS, Jackson DC: The role of the radiologist in acute gastrointestinal bleeding. Gastrointest Radiol 3:357–368, 1978.
Oddson TA, Johnsrude IS Jr, Jackson DC, Rice RP: Acute gastrointestinal hemorrhage. The changing role of barium examinations. Radiol Clin North Am 16:123–133, 1978.
Thoeni RF, Cello JP: A critical look at the accuracy of endoscopy and double-contrast radiography of the upper gastrointestinal (UGI) tract in patients with substantial UGI hemorrhage. Radiology 135:305–308, 1980.

Trauma

Gould RJ, Thorwarth WT: Retroperitoneal rupture of the duodenum due to blunt non-penetrating abdominal trauma. Radiology 80:743, 1963.
Love L, Berkow AE: Trauma to the esophagus. Gastrointest Radiol 2:305–321, 1978.
McCort JJ: Intraperitoneal and retroperitoneal hemorrhage. Symposium on the alimentary tract. Radiol Clin North Am 14:391, 1976.

Contrast and the Emergency Patient

Cochran DQ, Almond CH, Shucart WA: An experimental study of the effects of barium and intestinal contents on the peritoneal cavity. Am J Roentgenol 89:883–887, 1963.
Jacobson G, Berne CJ, Meyers HI, Rosoff L: The examination of patients with suspected perforated ulcer using a water-soluble contrast medium. Am J Roentgenol 86:37–49, 1961.
Nelson SW, Christoforidis AJ: The use of barium sulfate suspensions in the study of suspected mechanical obstruction of the small intestine. Am J Roentgenol 101:367–378, 1967.
Seltzer SE, Jones B, McLaughlin GC: Proper choice of contrast agents in emergency gastrointestinal radiology. CRC Crit Rev Diagn Imaging 12:79, 1979.
Vassal K, Montali RJ, Larson SM, Chaffee V, James AE Jr: Evaluation of barium and Gastrografin as contrast media for the diagnosis of esophageal ruptures or perforations. Am J Roentgenol 123:307–319, 1975.

4

MOTILITY DISORDERS

Substances taken orally pass along the gastrointestinal tract propelled by wavelike muscular contractions (peristalsis). These waves are responsible for the smoothly undulating appearance of the bowel and account for the changing appearance of the bowel from film to film. Observing peristalsis is an integral part of the examination of the pharynx, esophagus, and stomach but plays less role in the study of the remainder of the gastrointestinal tract. This is especially true in air contrast work, when the bowel is paralyzed. Occasionally peristalsis may cause problems during a study; during a barium enema, persistent contraction (spasm) may result in premature evacuation of the barium.

Illustrating a dynamic process such as peristalsis with words and static images is very difficult, but first we will describe normal peristalsis in different organs and note how disease may produce abnormal peristalsis or motility. In general, if a disease process affects muscle itself or the neural supply to that muscle, a motility disorder will result.

PHARYNGEAL MOTILITY

The pharynx is often neglected by radiologists and may not even be examined at all during a routine UGI series, an unfortunate omission. It must, however, be observed more carefully than usual in any patient who complains of swallowing or choking problems.

Swallowing involves a series of extremely complex movements, requiring sophisticated coordination among tongue, palate, and pharynx. These movements are extremely rapid and to study them adequately either cineradiography or videotape recording is necessary.

The muscle of the pharynx is *striated* muscle; therefore, any disease that involves striated muscle, e.g., myasthenia gravis or dermatomyositis, or affects the neural supply to these muscles (cranial nerves IX, X, and XII) may result in a swallowing abnormality.

The tongue transfers the bolus to the back of the mouth. Three structures are particularly important in maintaining normal pharyngeal function: the uvula, the epiglottis, and the cricopharyngeus muscle. The uvula must appose the posterior pharyngeal wall to prevent regurgitation of food into the nose; the epiglottis must cover the entrance to the larynx to prevent aspiration (Fig. 4–1); and the cricopharyngeus must relax at the appropriate time to allow the bolus to pass. Since the pharynx rises a significant distance during swallowing, scarring or fibrosis around the pharynx limiting this elevation may also result in abnormality.

Common findings in pharyngeal disease include the following: (1) dilatation of the hypopharynx at rest; (2) incoordinate fluttering movements of the tongue; (3) reflux of food (or barium) into the nasopharynx (Fig. 4–2); (4) failure to empty the valleculae and pyriform fossae completely with each swallow; and (5) aspiration into the larynx.

A number of motility abnormalities may occur at the *pharyngoesophageal* junction. Nor-

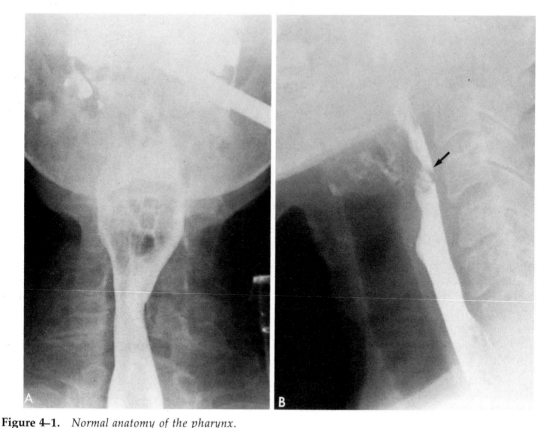

Figure 4–1. *Normal anatomy of the pharynx.*
A, Frontal view of the normal pharynx, distended by barium.
B, Normal lateral view of the pharynx. The bolus is distending the pharynx and cervical esophagus. The epiglottis (arrow) has flipped down to cover the entrance to the larynx.

mally, the cricopharyngeus muscle (situated at the level of C5-6) should relax to allow the bolus to pass into the esophagus. Incoordination of relaxation of this muscle, with contraction of the rest of the pharynx, results in what is known as *pharyngeal dysmotility* ("cricopharyngeal achalasia"). Some surgeons would advise a myotomy in this condition, but the results have been somewhat disappointing.

Zenker's diverticulum (Fig. 4–3), a pulsion diverticulum, occurs at the pharyngoesophageal junction through a potentially weak area posteriorly (the crossing of the oblique and horizontal fibers of the constrictor muscle). Abnormal peristalsis may cause herniation through this weak area, resulting in a diverticulum. The precise manner in which these form is still speculative, but because most of these people have abnormal esophageal motility and gross reflux, these are thought to play some role. When small, these diverticula always point backwards, but as they become bigger, they will flop to one side

or the other; sometimes the diagnosis can be made on plain films by seeing an air-fluid level in the neck. The patient may complain of regurgitating undigested food eaten a day or days before. Occasionally these diverticula may become so large that obstruction of the esophagus results and overflow aspiration occurs.

Cervical webs are usually found on the anterior wall of the esophagus below the cricopharyngeus. A web may consist purely of mucosa or may be a fibrous band that partially or almost completely blocks the esophagus. Webs may be seen only when the esophagus is fully distended and may not be visible when only small sips of barium are taken. Characteristically dysphagia due to webs will be cured by endoscopy. Webs have been associated with iron deficiency anemia (Plummer-Vinson or Paterson-Kelly syndrome, depending from which side of the Atlantic one comes from), and perhaps an increased risk of developing esophageal cancer. Webs are uncom-

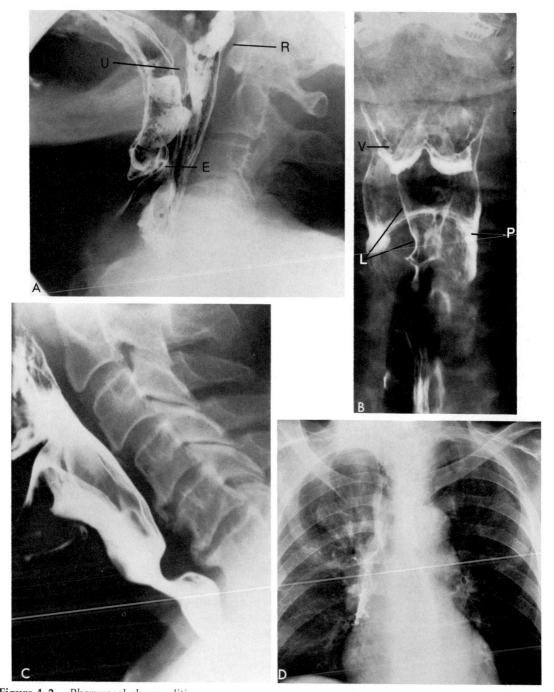

Figure 4–2. *Pharyngeal abnormalities.*

A, Reflux into the nasopharynx. The uvula (*U*) has failed to appose the posterior pharyngeal wall and barium (*R*) has "refluxed" up into the nasal passages. Barium is also coating the *under*surface of the epiglottis (*E*), and there is a small amount of barium dribbling into the larynx.

B, Aspiration. A barium (not Gastrografin!) swallow shows aspiration into the larynx. Barium is outlining not only the valleculae (*V*) and pyriform sinuses (*P*), but also the larynx (*L*) and trachea, indicating aspiration. Note the retained barium in the valleculae, another sign of pharyngeal dysfunction.

C, Aspiration due to pharyngeal dysmotility ("cricopharyngeal achalasia"). On this lateral film from a barium swallow, there is a small amount of contrast material on the undersurface of the epiglottis entering the larynx; the epiglottis has not flipped down adequately to prevent aspiration. Note the large thumb-shaped filling defect posteriorly at the level of C5-6, which is the cricopharyngeus muscle; this has failed to relax at the appropriate time to allow the bolus to pass by. Incidentally, note the degenerative change in the cervical spine.

D, Chest x-ray of same patient as in *B* demonstrating *aspiration* into the bronchial tree. Note the infiltrate in the right upper lobe, which was due to chronic aspiration pneumonia.

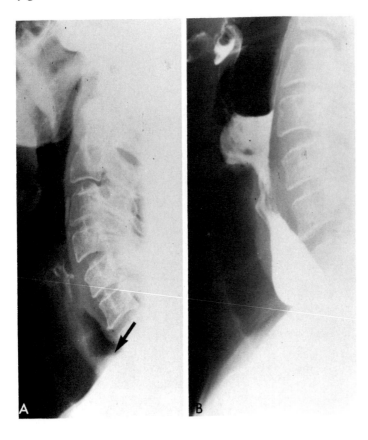

Figure 4–3. *Zenker's diverticulum. A,* This lateral film shows an air-fluid level projected over the prevertebral soft tissues (arrow) owing to fluid within the diverticulum. *B,* Following administration of contrast medium, the cause of the air-fluid level is evident, a large Zenker's diverticulum. The pharynx is dilated and there is another air-fluid level within it due to partial obstruction by the diverticulum.

mon; do not overdiagnose them. One must not confuse the normal triangular defect on the anterior wall of the esophagus (postcricoid impression) with a web (a horizontal linear filling defect).

EXAMINATION OF THE PHARYNX. Motility itself can best be observed with the patient in the lateral position, but, as with any contrast study, a preliminary film (soft tissue technique) of the neck should be obtained and vocal cord movement checked fluoroscopically. Swallowing is then observed in the lateral position for several swallows and abnormalities such as regurgitation into the nose, aspiration, and so forth, watched for carefully. If there is concern that the patient may aspirate, use barium. The patient will not be adversely affected if he aspirates thin barium, as barium is inert in the lung. As stated previously, water-soluble contrast medium is strongly contraindicated in any patient who may aspirate (patient coughs when he swallows) or who may have a fistula (e.g., tracheoesophageal) into the lung.

If aspiration does occur, it is necessary to find out why the patient is aspirating. Is it because of a motility disturbance? Is there a distal obstruction with "overflow aspiration"? Is the cause in fact not aspiration at all but a tracheoesophageal fistula? Surprisingly, it can at times be difficult to differentiate between a high fistula and aspiration. A small feeding tube may then be placed in the esophagus and contrast medium (barium or oily Dionosil) injected while withdrawing the tube until a fistula is either confirmed or excluded.

ESOPHAGEAL MOTILITY

Esophageal motility is much slower than pharyngeal motility and can readily be observed fluoroscopically. Peristaltic waves in the esophagus are of three types:

PRIMARY STRIPPING WAVE. The *primary stripping wave* is initiated by swallowing and actively strips the esophagus of its contents. Each stripping wave is preceded by a negative wave, which results in relaxation of the gastroesophageal junction (cardia) to accept the bolus.

SECONDARY STRIPPING WAVE. Anything not removed from the esophagus by the primary stripping wave is cleared by a *secondary stripping wave*, which is stimulated by distention and begins at the level of the remaining bolus.

TERTIARY CONTRACTIONS. Both primary and secondary waves are propulsive, but there are also nonpropulsive, uncoordinated waves (*tertiary contractions*), which increase with age and are usually not of clinical significance.

Many abnormalities of esophageal motility may occur, the most common being (1) absent or poor primary stripping wave, e.g., in *scleroderma*, or secondary to reflux esophagitis, presbyesophagus; (2) failure of the gastroesophageal sphincter to relax to accept the bolus, i.e., *achalasia*; (3) simultaneous contraction of tertiary waves, resulting in a form of esophageal spasm, the *"corkscrew esophagus"* (Fig. 4–4). Esophageal spasm is important because it may cause "atypical chest pain;" the radiologist will be asked many times about esophageal motility in patients with this clinical syndrome. More confusion with angina may arise clinically because esophageal spasm may also relax with nitroglycerin. The ability to produce esophageal spasm with an acid barium mixture has been used as a provocative test for reflux esophagitis; an inflamed esophagus may be acutely sensitive to acid barium and may either go into spasm or become aperistaltic on contact with it, whereas a normal esophagus is unaffected.

Peristalsis should be observed with the patient lying down. It is important to remember that true peristalsis can be assessed only in the horizontal position. In the erect position, what appears to be a stripping wave is in fact the esophagus collapsing behind the bolus; if the gastroesophageal junction functions normally, the esophagus empties purely by gravity in the erect position. To watch the primary wave, ask the patient to swallow one (and only one) mouthful of barium; the primary stripping wave should pass all the way into the stomach. If the patient misunderstands you

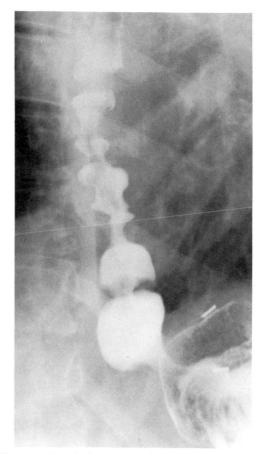

Figure 4–4. *Corkscrew esophagus.* Multiple indentations due to deep tertiary contractions give a corkscrew appearance to the esophagus.

and keeps on drinking, the primary wave will be interrupted but can be observed on the *last* swallow, when the patient stops drinking.

If there is a poor stripping wave, two major conditions must be differentiated — i.e., scleroderma and achalasia — both of which will result in a dilated esophagus and the absence of a stripping wave (Table 4–1). Since these two diseases affect the gastroesophageal junction differently, they can usually be distinguished by fluoroscopy in both the erect and horizontal positions.

ACHALASIA. *Achalasia*, a disease of young people, affects primarily the gastroesophageal junction, which fails to relax with each swallow as it should; this is due to degeneration of Auerbach's plexus. It will relax (although not completely) only when the hydrostatic pressure of a column of food or

TABLE 4–1. DIFFERENTIATION OF SCLERODERMA AND ACHALASIA

	Scleroderma	Achalasia
Esophagus	Mildly dilated	Massively dilated
Gastroesophageal junction	Wide open	Closed (tapers to a cigar shape)
Erect	Empties by gravity	Maintains air-fluid level No fundic air bubble
Horizontal	No stripping wave	No stripping wave
Reflux	Yes Associated hiatus hernia common, eventually results in stricture	No (may occur after Heller myotomy)

liquid overcomes the increased pressure in the lower esophageal "sphincter," after which the esophagus will empty in spurts. In the horizontal position, the esophagus will not empty at all.

Owing to the functional distal obstruc-tion, the esophagus in achalasia will dilate progressively and eventually overflow aspiration may occur, with recurrent chest "infections." On chest x-ray a large paramediastinal mass and often an air-fluid level in the mediastinum will be seen (Fig. 4–5). Characteris-

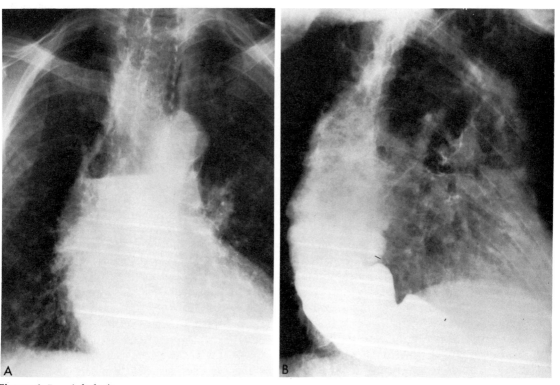

Figure 4–5. *Achalasia.*

A, On this erect chest film there is an air-fluid level in the mediastinum within a markedly dilated esophagus (remember the esophagus is a mediastinal organ). There are bilateral changes at the lung bases due to multiple episodes of aspiration.

B, This barium swallow demonstrates a markedly dilated and tortuous esophagus with retained particulate matter. Note how the distal esophagus tapers to a conical beak, a characteristic finding in achalasia.

tically, the gastric air bubble is absent. The incidence of esophageal carcinoma is increased in patients with achalasia, but tumors can be missed because they are hidden by food or other debris. Onset of achalasia-type symptoms in an older person requires particular attention, since cancer of the gastroesophageal junction may mimic the symptoms and radiologic findings of this disease. In South America, a trypanosomal infection (Chagas' disease) is indistinguishable from idiopathic achalasia. The motility of the remainder of the gastrointestinal tract in idiopathic achalasia is normal, but other organs may be affected in Chagas' disease.

SCLERODERMA. *Scleroderma*, one of the collagen-vascular diseases, involves smooth muscle and therefore affects the middle and distal thirds of the esophagus, sparing the pharynx. Any other part of the GI tract may be affected, resulting in poor motility, dilatation, and sacculation (or pseudodiverticula, which characteristically are eccentric and seen especially in the colon). Slow gastric emptying and slow small bowel transit times are common (Fig. 4–6), and there may be associated malabsorption due to stasis and bacterial overgrowth. The duodenum may become dilated and floppy (megaduodenum) and may become so massive that the superior mesenteric artery (SMA) syndrome may result.

Characteristically, so far as the esophagus is concerned, the gastroesophageal junction is wide open in scleroderma, so that in the erect position the esophagus will empty by gravity. In the horizontal position, however, peristalsis is absent and the esophagus remains filled. In addition, because the gastroesophageal junction is wide open, free reflux is common; resultant reflux esophagitis frequently leads to stricture formation.

Although usually patients with scleroderma will have peripheral signs and symptoms before gut manifestations, occasionally it will be the motility disturbance that will cause them to seek medical help. One should therefore think of scleroderma in patients with poor peristalsis, especially if it is associated with Raynaud's disease. Dilated atonic bowel with or without sacculation should also suggest this diagnosis.

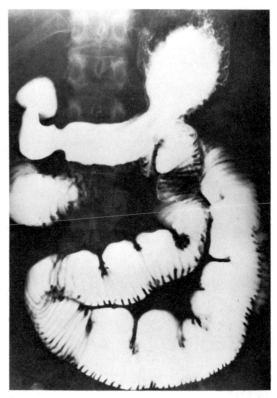

Figure 4–6. *Scleroderma.* This 90 minute film showing exceedingly slow transit time demonstrates markedly dilated bowel with eccentric pseudosacculations. The folds opposite the sacculations are normal.

Hiatus Hernia

Hiatus hernia is probably the most overdiagnosed "abnormality" on UGI series (Fig. 4–8). It results from weakening of the phrenicoesophageal ligaments or widening of the diaphragmatic hiatus (an aging process?) or both, and is aggravated by increased intra-abdominal pressure, which forces the stomach up into the chest (e.g., multiple pregnancies, constipation, and so forth).

There are two types of hiatus hernia, the sliding and the paraesophageal; each has different symptoms, methods of treatment, and prognosis. It is important, therefore, to differentiate between the two types of hernia, and this is done radiologically. In the sliding or axial type, the gastroesophageal junction has risen into the chest and is now above the diaphragm; the patient will complain of reflux symptoms as the antireflux mechanisms (hia-

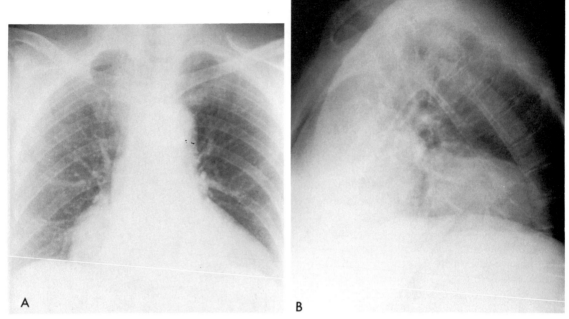

Figure 4–7. *Chest x-ray with mediastinal mass. A,* On the posteroanterior film, a mass is seen in the right cardiophrenic angle. *B,* On the lateral film this is seen to lie in the posterior mediastinum; a barium swallow demonstrated this to be a hiatus hernia. Occasionally, you will see an air-fluid level within the mass and then this diagnosis can be made on the plain film.

tal contraction, acute angle of submerged esophagus–stomach relationship) can no longer function. In a paraesophageal hernia, on the other hand, the gastroesophageal junction is in its normal position, but part of the stomach has herniated above the diaphragm to lie *next* (para) to the esophagus; this occurs either through the hiatus itself or through some other hole in the diaphragm. The patient with this type of hernia will not complain of reflux, and in fact often will have no complaints. He may develop a problem only if the hernia tries to descend back into the abdomen and becomes strangulated, an emergency situation.

A number of questions must therefore be asked regarding "hiatus hernia:" Is there a hernia? If so, what type of hernia is it? (Where is the gastroesophageal junction?) Is there gastroesophageal reflux?

One of the reasons why hernias are over-diagnosed is the existence of a normal saclike dilatation of the distal esophagus (the phrenic ampulla), and this is sometimes confused with a hernia. To diagnose a hernia, one must see either the *gastroesophageal junction* or gastric folds above the diaphragm. In the normal patient, another part of the esophagus will also be seen below the diaphragm — the so-called submerged or abdominal segment; this will not be seen in the patient with a hernia.

Another reason for the overdiagnosis of hiatus hernia may be explained by recent work of Whalen (personal communication), who believes that the hiatus actually lies a few centimeters above the apparent level of the diaphragm. Further work is necessary to clarify this controversy.

To help locate the gastroesophageal junction look for two rings in the distal esophagus, one of which is normal, one of which means there is a hernia. These rings are known as the A (Wolf) and the B (Schatzki) rings (Fig. 4–8). The A ring is a normal finding and merely represents the region of lower esophageal sphincter (LES). Remember, there is no true anatomic sphincter in the lower esophagus; the LES is merely an area 2 to 3 cm long in which the intraluminal pressure is higher than in the adjacent esophagus. The B ring (otherwise known as the Z-line) is the actual squamocolumnar junction between esophagus and stomach. If *this* ring is seen above the diaphragm, ipso facto a hernia is present. The characteristics of these two rings differ. Various maneuvers that raise the intra-abdominal pressure are used to "bring out" a hernia or B ring, e.g., swallowing over a bolster and straining following repetitive swallows. Many people have hernias and most are not clinically significant; the ones that may be are those with associated reflux, because then there will be superimposed reflux esophagitis. The presence of a hernia is not as important as how easily acid can pass from the stomach into the esophagus. It is important to check for

reflux in all patients with a sliding hernia; reflux may be seen even without a hernia if the hiatus is patulous. It should be stressed that reflux is acid (or barium), which passes from the hernia back into the esophagus and not from the main body of the stomach into the hernia. The patient should be placed so that barium is in the fundus (or hernia), so that reflux can be seen more easily. Then various maneuvers to raise intra-abdominal pressure are performed, including coughing, straining, and leg-raising. Free reflux is even more significant; it is unprovoked and is seen as the patient turns from side to side. A swallow of cold water (the "water siphon" test) may result in a significant amount of

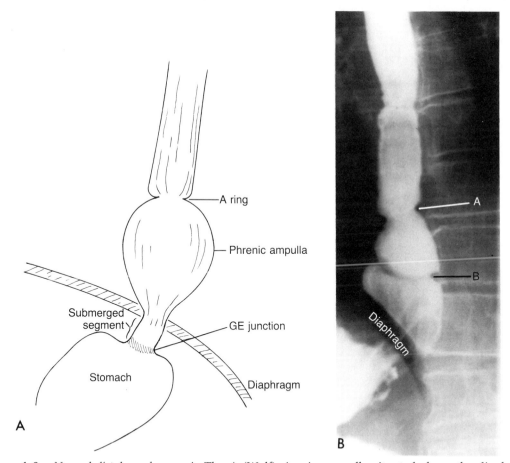

Figure 4–8. *Normal distal esophagus. A,* The A (Wolf) ring is normally situated above the diaphragm. Below it, the esophagus widens and appears saccular, the phrenic ampulla, another normal finding. Below the diaphragm is another part of the esophagus, the submerged segment. *B,* Compare this appearance with the findings in a small hiatus hernia. There are now two rings, the A and B rings. Note their different appearance; the proximal (A) has a rounded appearance, the distal (B) appears squared off. Note the gastric folds crossing the diaphragm, confirming that this is a hernia.

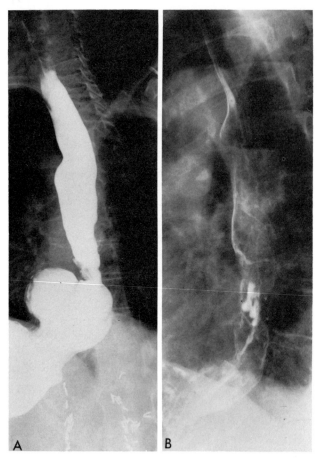

A

B

Figure 4–9. *A, Esophagitis.* There is a large hiatus hernia with proximal esophageal dilatation, and narrowing and irregularity in the distal few centimeters of the esophagus. The narrowing is a stricture and the irregularity suggests esophagitis.

B, Esophagitis with ulcerations. Even a suboptimal air contrast study demonstrates that there are multiple pools of contrast medium within the strictured area in the distal esophagus consistent with acute ulcerations. Note that in the presence of active inflammation, it can at times be difficult to differentiate between esophagitis and a malignancy. Endoscopy and biopsy may be necessary.

Figure 4–10. *Barrett's esophagus.* In the upper third of the esophagus, there is a stricture with a projection posteriorly consistent with an ulcer crater. A biopsy showed columnar epithelium–lined esophagus.

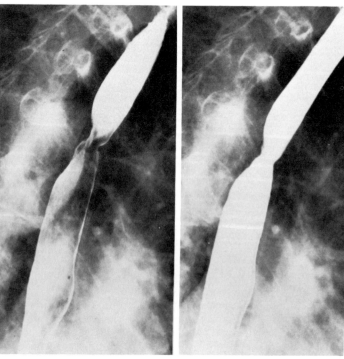

barium reflux; many people say that this test correlates well with clinical symptoms of reflux esophagitis.

Acid reflux into the esophagus results in esophagitis (see Chapter 6) with a spectrum of radiographic findings from spasm to ulceration and eventual stricture (Fig. 4–9). When a stricture has formed, symptoms will change from those of reflux and irritability (heartburn) to dysphagia. A barium tablet of known diameter (1.25 cm) is useful in assessing the diameter of a stricture.

Another change may take place in the esophagus as the result of long-standing reflux, the columnar epithelium–lined or Barrett esophagus (Fig. 4–10). The normal squamous epithelium of the esophagus is progressively transformed into columnar epithelium. Originally this was thought to be the result of congenital islands of gastric mucosa in the esophagus, but it is now known that this is an acquired condition due to chronic reflux. It is important to be aware of this entity because it is associated with an increased incidence of esophageal cancer. The appearance varies, but a stricture or ulceration high up in the esophagus should suggest this diagnosis, especially if associated with reflux or a hernia. Following antireflux surgery, the epithelium may regress to normal.

Other causes of esophagitis, e.g., candidiasis, herpes, radiation, lye ingestion, produce an appearance very similar to reflux esophagitis (but without the hernia). The finding of plaques (filling defects) or linear ulcers may suggest Candida as the cause. Acute esophagitis due to ingestion of irritant substances tends to be maximal at points of holdup, such as the aortic arch.

GASTRIC MOTILITY

Gastric emptying depends upon many things, including how hot or cold the food is, how big the meal, how much carbohydrate, fat, and protein it contains, and how relaxed or anxious the person is. One of the most common causes of delayed gastric emptying is fear or anxiety. "Pylorospasm" is a common annoyance during the performance of a GI

series; it may be overcome simply by talking with the patient (asking such questions as "what's your favorite food?"), by giving more barium, and sometimes by having the patient breathe deeply. Delayed gastric emptying may also be due to organic disease at the gastric outlet (e.g., a pyloric channel ulcer, antral carcinoma), or it may indicate abnormal motility, as in diabetes. Naturally in chronic outlet obstruction, secretions will be retained in the stomach, and a poor-quality examination of the remainder of the stomach is to be expected.

Many drugs, such as morphine, will delay gastric emptying. Sometimes these drugs can be put to use in radiology; glucagon is given during an air contrast UGI series to abolish peristalsis. Another drug, metoclopramide (Reglan), is used widely in Europe to speed gastric emptying in patients with pylorospasm and will also speed small bowel series. Basically, however, if the stomach will not empty, the question is — is the problem merely pylorospasm or is it disease?

Gastric peristalsis may be observed if glucagon has not been given. Peristalsis will pass through a benign lesion but will be interrupted by a malignancy. Propulsive peristalsis tends to begin at the angularis and progresses through the antrum on both greater and lesser curvatures to the pylorus. Occasionally these waves may be so deep that pseudoulcers are created (see Chapter 11). If glucagon has abolished peristalsis, one should observe instead whether all areas of the stomach are distensible and pliable. If a nonperistaltic area is pliable, it is unlikely to represent a malignancy, which instead would be rigid. The gloved hand should be used to palpate suspicious areas.

Vagotomy delays gastric emptying, and a concurrent drainage procedure is necessary (pyloroplasty, gastroenterostomy). Markedly delayed emptying may be a problem immediately postvagotomy, but this will usually subside in a few weeks. Other postvagotomy problems include an achalasia-like syndrome, dumping, diarrhea, small bowel dilatation, and even unmasking of sprue. The gallbladder is also affected, with poor contraction, a change in the chemical composition of the bile itself, and possibly an increased incidence of gallstones. All these effects are less when highly selective vagotomy has been performed than with truncal vagotomy.

COLONIC MOTILITY

Colonic motor contractions are of three main types: (1) *tonic*, which maintain resting tone, (2) *nonpropulsive localized contractions*, involving either a short segment or only a single haustrum, and (3) *propulsive mass peristalsis*, which propels the fecal stream along.

Localized segmental contractions may be seen during the barium enema, and these may cause cramping. There are specific areas in the colon where these are more common, and they may be confused with pathologic findings (see Chapter 11). Colonic distention by the enema may stimulate these segmental contractions, with resultant spasm. Wait until these areas relax before proceeding, or give an antispasmodic, e.g., glucagon. In certain groups of patients, as, for example, those with irritable bowel, inflammatory bowel disease, and diverticulosis, there may be much more spasm, and in these patients the routine use of glucagon is helpful. Continuing to run in barium when the colon is in spasm will result in the patient's "blowing the enema." Anxiety alone produces spasm, and the enema should be performed in a relaxed and supportive atmosphere. Whether a lot of spasm can be equated with abnormality, however, is debatable. Certainly whether it indicates "spastic colitis" or "irritable bowel syndrome" is doubtful; in fact, many would not call these radiologic diagnoses at all.

Diverticula

Pulsion diverticula are found at points of weakness in the bowel wall. The diverticula in the colon are of the pulsion type; the weak point is where the nutrient arteries penetrate the wall. The most common other site for a pulsion diverticulum is in the neck, where Zenker's diverticulum, which has already been discussed, is found.

A traction diverticulum, on the other hand, is formed when the wall of the bowel becomes adherent to an adjacent inflammatory process and continuing peristalsis causes an outpouching. The most common site for this to occur is at the carina adjacent to diseased hilar lymph nodes.

Other diverticula may be (1) epiphrenic (do not confuse it with a paraesophageal hernia), (2) gastric (usually high on the lesser curvature near the gastroesophageal junction), (3) inner aspect of the duodenal C-sweep, and (4) jejunal (if multiple, they may be associated with stasis and resulting malabsorption). Occasionally, a diverticulum might be confused with an ulcer, but the lack of spasm and the presence of mucosa within the diverticulum should suggest the correct diagnosis.

A congenital (and therefore true) diverticulum is the Meckel's diverticulum, which follows the "rule-of-two's": 2 inches long; male-to-female ratio, 2/1; located 2 feet from the ileocecal valve, and present in 2 per cent of the population. It contains gastric mucosa approximately 20 per cent of the time and therefore may bleed or ulcerate. Although present in 2 per cent of people at autopsy, a Meckel's diverticulum is very rarely demonstrated on a small bowel series. This is because, unlike acquired diverticula, it does contain a muscle layer; if it fills, contraction and peristalsis will promptly empty it of any barium. Characteristically, acquired diverticula remain filled with barium for a prolonged period of time.

Diverticulosis

In general, by the term "diverticulosis" is meant multiple colonic diverticula. Many theories have been proposed to account for the development of diverticulosis, a disease of Western civilization often attributed to a diet deficient in fiber. However, an abnormality in motility, i.e., a hypercontracted segment in which the intraluminal pressure is extremely high, has been found in both constipated individuals and in patients with diverticulosis. Diverticula may occur anywhere in the colon but are most common in the sigmoid colon, where the intraluminal pressure is

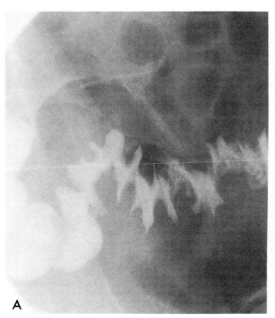 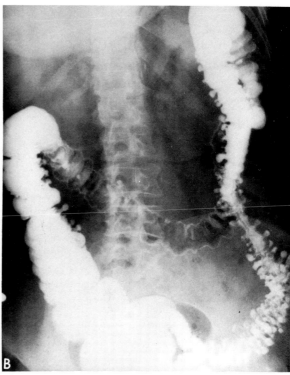

Figure 4–11. *A, Muscular hypertrophy in prediverticulosis.* Marked hypertrophy of the muscle in the sigmoid colon gives a sawtoothed appearance to this segment. *B, Diverticulosis.* Multiple rounded outpouchings paralleling the colon are diverticula; these occur at the sites where the vessels penetrate the wall.

highest (Fig. 4–11). Muscular hypertrophy is part of the pathology, resulting in spasm and a sawtoothed appearance. The effect of the raised intraluminal pressure is maximal at points of weakness (where the nutrient artery penetrates the wall). At these points, outpouchings of mucosa through the muscular layer will develop, with the formation of false diverticula.

Complications include bleeding and perforation. It has been said that left-sided diverticula tend to perforate and right-sided ones to bleed. This is a generalization, of course, because those in the cecum become inflamed and sigmoid diverticula certainly do bleed, sometimes massively. Free perforation is uncommon in diverticulitis; the perforation is usually sealed off to form an abscess. Free perforation is more likely to occur in patients with poor defense mechanisms.

Diverticulitis has already been discussed in Chapter 3, so the x-ray findings will merely be summarized here. Spasm and muscular hypertrophy are part of the process of diverticulosis and do not by themselves mean diverticulitis. The perforation or evidence of abscess formation must be seen on the radiograph. Extravasation of contrast medium or a mass effect must likewise be seen. A postevacuation film is extremely important in suspected diverticulitis, because extravasation may be demonstrated only after the bowel has actively contracted.

References

General

Seaman WB: Motor dysfunction of the gastrointestinal tract; Hickey Lecture, 1972. Am J Roentgenol 116:235–244, 1972.
Silver TM, Farber SJ, Bole GG, Martel W: Radiologic features of mixed connective tissue disease and scleroderma–systemic lupus erythematosus overlap. Radiology 120:269–276, 1976.
Simpson AJ, Khilnani MT: Gastrointestinal manifestations of the muscular dystrophies: A review of roentgen findings. Am J Roentgenol 125:948–955, 1975.
Udoff EJ, Genant HK, Kozin F, Ginsberg M: Mixed connective

tissue disease: The spectrum of radiographic manifestations. Radiology 124:613–618, 1977.

Esophagus

Cho KJ, Hunter TB, Whitehouse WM: The columnar epithelial–lined lower esophagus and its association with adenocarcinoma of the esophagus. Radiology 115:563–568, 1975.

Clements JL Jr, Cox GW, Torres WE, Weens HS: Cervical esophageal webs — a roentgen-anatomic correlation. Am J Roentgenol 121:221–231, 1974.

Diseases of the pharynx and larynx. Curr Probl Diagn Radiol, Vol. 7, 1977.

Dodds WJ: 1976 Walter B Cannon Lecture: current concepts of esophageal motor function: clinical implications for radiology. Am J Roentgenol 128:549–563, 1977.

Friedland GW: Progress in radiology: Historical review of the changing concepts of lower esophageal anatomy: 430 BC –1977. Am J Roentgenol 131:373–388, 1978.

Margulis AR, Koehler RE: Radiologic diagnosis of disordered esophageal motility: A unified physiologic approach. Radiol Clin North Am 14:429–439, 1976.

Nosher JL, Campbell WL, Seaman WB: The clinical significance of cervical esophageal and hypopharyngeal webs. Radiology 117:45–47, 1975.

Olmsted WW, Madewell JE: The esophageal and small-bowel manifestations of progressive systemic sclerosis. A pathophysiologic explanation of the roentgenographic signs. Gastrointest Radiol 1:33–36, 1976.

Ott DJ, Gelfand DW, Wu WC: Reflux esophagitis: radiographic and endoscopic correlation. Radiology 130:583–588, 1979.

Palmer ED: Disorders of the cricopharyngeus muscle: A review. Gastroenterology 71:510–519, 1976.

The pharynx and larynx. Semin Roentgenol 9:253–323, 1974.

Robbins AH, Hermos JA, Schimmel EM, Friedlander DM, Messian RA: The columnar lined esophagus — analysis of 26 cases. Radiology 123:1–7, 1977.

Wolf BS: Sliding hiatal hernia: The need for redefinition. Am J Roentgenol 117:231–246, 1973.

Wolf BS: The inferior esophageal sphincter — anatomic, roentgenologic and manometric correlation, contraindications, and terminology. Am J Roentgenol 110:260, 1970.

Stomach

Donner MW: Normal and abnormal motility of the stomach. Radiol Clin North Am 14:441–460, 1976.

Gramm HF, Reuter K, Costello P: The radiologic manifestations of diabetic gastric neuropathy and its differential diagnosis. Gastrointest Radiol 3:151–156, 1978.

Colon

Bryk D, Soong KY: Colonic ileus and its differential roentgen diagnosis. Am J Roentgenol 101:329–337, 1967.

Meyers MA: Colonic ileus. Gastrointest Radiol 2:37–40, 1977.

Peptic ulcer disease is so common that most general radiologists will study patients daily to confirm or exclude ulcer disease. A thorough appreciation of this important topic is vital from the very beginning of radiologic training.

Although there are important etiologic and clinical distinctions between duodenal and gastric ulcers, pathologically and radiologically the processes and end results are similar, so ulceration can be discussed abstractly before applying the concepts to specific clinical entities. Pathologically, an ulcer is an erosive process involving at least mucosa, usually submucosa, and often muscularis, and occasionally extending through all layers, resulting in perforation. The end result is a depression or hole in the lining of the gut, analogous to a well. If barium or any contrast medium is poured into the well, it will fill and an additional shadow (i.e., the collection of barium) will be visualized on the x-ray. An ulcer will appear as a pool of barium regardless of the organ in which it occurs.

PEPTIC ULCERS

As stated, ulcers can occur in any GI tract organ when the mucosa is damaged. In this chapter, classic peptic ulcer disease and its effects on stomach and duodenum will be described. Certain generalizations about peptic disease are worth noting before discussing the radiology of ulcers. The disease tends to be a disease of developed society, affects men

more than women, and is exacerbated by drugs such as alcohol and nicotine. Duodenal ulcers are the most common and are invariably benign, whereas only 95 per cent of gastric ulcers are benign; 5 per cent of them occur in malignancies. Obviously many more duodenal ulcers will be seen by you as a radiologist but what really counts is to distinguish between benign and malignant *gastric* ulcers.

RADIOLOGIC APPEARANCE OF ULCERS

The radiologist's purpose is twofold: (1) to find the ulcer, and (2) to decide whether it is benign or malignant.

The first task, to find the ulcer, is frequently more difficult than it may seem. Radiologists are certainly less than 100 per cent accurate in finding ulcers; 80 per cent would be a reasonable figure (less if the patient has active bleeding). Occasionally this is because the ulcer crater is too superficial (it just does not hold enough barium to be noticeable), too small (air contrast techniques are helpful here), or even too large (incredible as it may sound, it is sometimes harder to see a huge ulcer than a smaller one).

In order to visualize an ulcer crater, it must be filled with contrast medium (for an exception, see later discussion of double contrast examination) and highlighted from the opaque barium background by positioning or compression, or both. There are two ways a crater may be seen: *en face* (looking directly down into the well) or *in profile* (with the ulcer viewed from the side). En face, a typical ulcer crater will be a distinct round, circumscribed collection of barium; in profile the collection will again be distinct, but flatter. The collection will always have roughly the same shape because it is simply a hole filled with barium. An ulcer crater, or niche as it is sometimes called, is therefore a well-circumscribed, unchanging collection of barium reproducible from film to film at different times. during the examination. This point is important and should permit differentiation of a bona fide ulcer from diverticula or even collections of barium trapped between thickened folds.

If every ulcer could be seen in profile there would be no difficulty in finding them. Unfortunately, some ulcers cannot be profiled and must be searched for en face. The student may wonder how it is possible to find the small barium collection of the ulcer en face within a stomach full of opaque barium. This is why compression is so important. With compression the overlying barium collection is thinned enough to see the crater as a pool within a larger pool of barium (that is, as a double density). If compression is not performed, the ulcer may be missed entirely. If the ulcer is surrounded by sufficient edema, it may stand out more clearly, but compression is usually necessary for good visualization (Fig. 5–1).

When performing a double contrast examination, on the other hand, it is possible to demonstrate an *empty* ulcer crater whose rim has just been coated with barium. In this instance, the crater viewed en face will appear as a ring rather than a filled-in circle.

Once the radiologist has discovered an ulcer, he must decide if it is benign or malig-

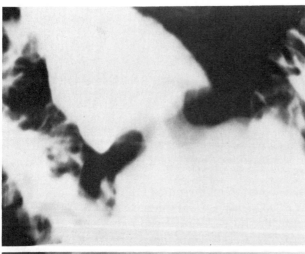
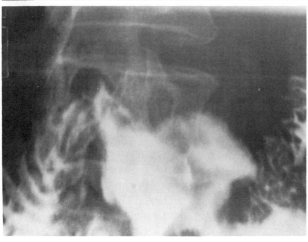

Figure 5–1. *Duodenal ulcer shown only with compression.* The upper film shows a normally shaped duodenal bulb without any evidence of ulceration. With compression, a central linear collection (an ulcer crater) with radiating folds is seen, and there is a surrounding filling defect indicating the edema mound. Without compression, this bulb would have been called normal.

nant. This applies primarily to gastric ulcers. There are a number of criteria that help in making this decision.

CRITERIA FOR BENIGNITY OF GASTRIC ULCERS

RADIATION OF FOLDS. Radiation of gastric folds right up to the ulcer crater indicates a benign ulcer. Cancers destroy and amputate folds for some distance around the ulcerated mass, and therefore the folds appear to stop abruptly well short of the crater. Occasionally, a tremendous edema mound surrounds a benign ulcer, simulating fold cut-off, so other criteria must also be relied upon.

PENETRATION OF ULCER CRATER BEYOND THE LUMEN. When viewed in profile, a benign ulcer will be seen to penetrate beyond the expected margin of the lumen. An ulcer in a malignancy will appear to lie within the lumen rather than penetrate the wall, because it lies within an intraluminal mass.

HAMPTON'S LINE. If a benign ulcer is radiographed precisely at right angles, a thin (1 to 2 mm), lucent line will occasionally be visible, which is caused by undamaged mucosa overhanging the crater mouth. This occurs because the submucosa is digested more rapidly, *undermining* the mucosa and leaving a thin veil at the crater mouth.

ULCER COLLAR. Moderately edematous tissue at the ulcer mouth produces a lucent mound when seen in profile.

ULCER MOUND. A large amount of edema surrounding an ulcer produces a lucent mound, especially when seen in profile. Both the collar and the mound can be large enough to simulate a mass. The smooth, obtuse junction with normal tissue distinguishes them from a tumor.

INCISURA. *Indrawing* of the wall opposite the ulcer (incisura) is a sign of a benign ulcer (Fig. 5–2).

PERISTALSIS. Peristalsis should continue normally through the region of the ulcer, and the area should be pliable.

MISCELLANEOUS. Some authors report ulcer shape as a helpful clue — a round, sharply circumscribed ulcer suggests benigni-

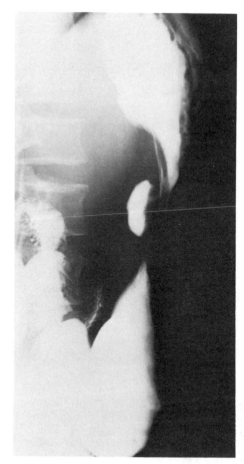

Figure 5–2. *Benign lesser curvature ulcer.* There is a large barium collection projecting beyond the expected line of the stomach, with folds radiating up to the ulcer itself. Note the inward deformity of the wall opposite the ulcer (the incisura).

ty. Most recent reports have stated that size and location are *not* helpful in distinguishing benign from malignant ulcers. In fact, some of the largest ulcers encountered, especially the giant gastric ulcers of the elderly, are benign.

CRITERIA FOR MALIGNANCY OF GASTRIC ULCERS

First, a semantic point should be cleared up — an ulcer per se is not malignant; a "malignant" ulcer is one that arises within a neoplasm that has outgrown its blood supply and become necrotic.

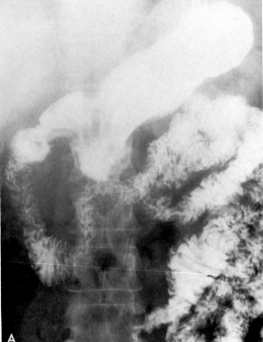

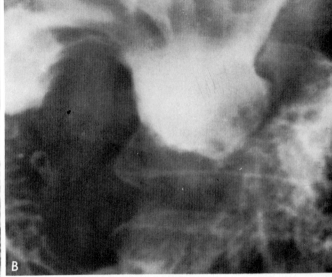

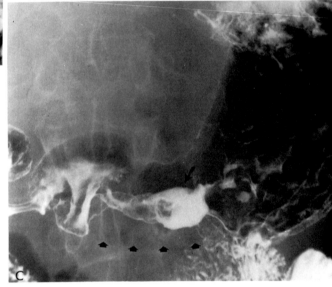

Figure 5–3. *Comparison of a benign ulcer and an ulcerating malignancy.* There is a very large projection from the greater curvature *(A)* and a coned-down view *(B)* shows that the folds radiate to the edge of the ulcer crater. Compare this appearance with *C*, in which there is a large irregular mass within the lumen, with a central ulceration (arrow). When the expected outline of the stomach is completed (arrowheads), the mass and ulcer clearly lie within the stomach and do not project out, as would a benign ulcer.

INTRALUMINAL LOCATION OF CRATER. Since a tumor mass is intraluminal, any ulceration that develops within this mass will appear to be located within the lumen of the stomach. Put another way, in malignant tumors, penetration through the wall away from the lumen is not demonstrated (Fig. 5–3C).

AMPUTATION OF FOLDS. An infiltrating tumor will destroy folds around the crater so that the folds stop short of the ulcer. Sometimes the folds are clubbed or otherwise abnormal in shape.

MISCELLANEOUS. Irregularly shaped craters with pointed margins suggest malignancy. Nodularity of surrounding mucosa is an ominous sign. The abrupt transition between tumor mound and normal stomach is in contrast to the smooth, obtuse margin between the edema mound of a benign ulcer and normal tissue.

Note should be made of an infrequently observed and poorly understood sign described by Carman and popularized by others, notably Kirklin. Carman's sign refers to a special type of flat carcinoma whose ulcer appears convex toward the lumen when it is compressed at fluoroscopy. (see Fig. 7–19.)

Applying the foregoing criteria, the radiologist should describe gastric ulcers as definitely benign, definitely malignant, or indeterminate. Endoscopy and biopsy should be encouraged for all except definitely benign ulcers; some advocate this approach for all gastric ulcers. Even if they appear benign, all gastric ulcers should be followed to *complete* healing by some modality, usually UGI series (Fig. 5–4). It should be stressed that *complete* healing must be demonstrated. Even ulcers in malignancies can become smaller following medical therapy; likewise, some benign ulcers can heal very slowly. However, an ulcer which

is *not* healing on a strict medical regimen must be suspected of being malignant and biopsied promptly.

DUODENAL ULCERS

Duodenal ulcers usually occur in the bulb, but postbulbar ulcers occurring at, or just distal to, the apex of the bulb are a well-known concomitant of peptic disease. Ulcers occurring elsewhere in duodenum or jejunum should suggest a more virulent process, such as Zollinger-Ellison syndrome (see later discussion). Duodenal ulcers are benign, are related to acid hypersecretion, and frequently produce classic symptoms of epigastric pain

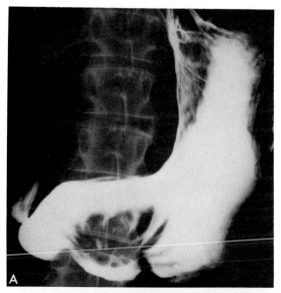

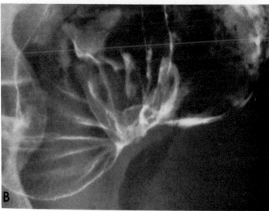

Figure 5–4. *Healing of giant gastric ulcer.*

A, A large ulcer crater with folds radiating all the way to it is seen. Sometimes on the greater curvature it may be difficult to differentiate between benign and malignant ulcers; even benign ulcers (as this was) may not appear to project as much as they do on the lesser curvature, so that one of the criteria of benignity sometimes cannot be applied.

B, Healing phase (not yet completely healed). There is still some mucosal irregularity and the folds are still radiating. With complete healing, the folds will still radiate, but to a point where there is no longer a central collection of barium.

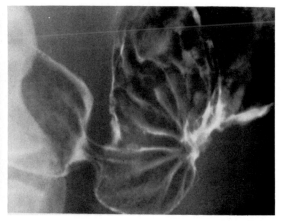

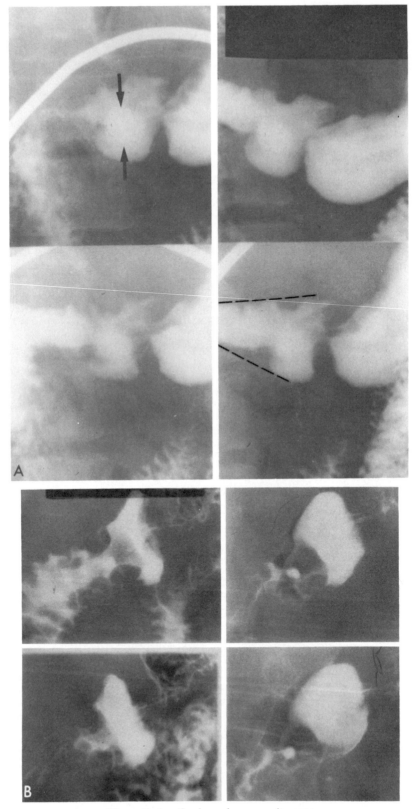

Figure 5–5. *See legend on opposite page*

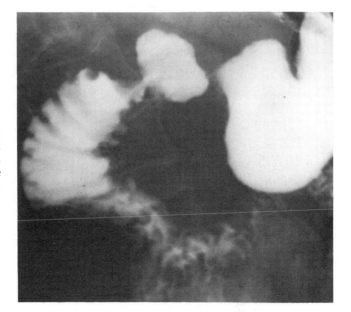

Figure 5–6. *Giant duodenal ulcer.* Although this collection of barium may appear at first glance to be the duodenal bulb, there was no change with peristalsis, and it did not empty, confirming that the entire bulb is now a giant ulcer. Note the antral pad sign and thickened folds in the descending duodenum.

between meals or pain that awakens the patient at night.

Demonstrating an ulcer in the bulb is similar to demonstrating one in the stomach (Fig. 5–5). A "niche" (constant, reproducible collection of barium) must be demonstrated and it is helpful to show folds radiating to the crater. It is imporant to remember that ulcers can occur on any wall of a viscus, and if the crater is not dependent, it will not fill with barium. For example, if a patient has an anterior wall ulcer and is examined only in the supine position without compression, it is possible that no barium will enter the crater and the ulcer will be missed.

Deformity associated with the crater is often more notable in the duodenal bulb than in the stomach. Marked indrawing of the bulb can occur, producing the so-called "cloverleaf" deformity; remember the ulcer is in the *center* of the cloverleaf. When the bulb is markedly deformed in this fashion, barium can collect in pseudodiverticula and between thickened folds, simulating an ulcer crater. A careful search for radiating folds and the persistence of the collection helps to distinguish a real ulcer from look-alikes (Fig. 5–9). Remember that deformity alone does not mean active disease: to diagnose active disease the ulcer niche must be found. Similarly, a normally shaped bulb does not exclude the presence of an ulcer; compression may bring out a shallow ulcer in a normal appearing bulb. Not all ulcers are round; they can be trenchlike and then will be linear collections rather than round ones (Fig. 5–7). These linear ulcers can occur de novo or during the healing phase of a typical round ulcer. Demonstrating the radiating fold pattern is particularly important in confirming the existence of a real crater. Interestingly, more deformity can be associated with linear ulcers than with regular round ulcers. Deformity of the bulb should alert the radiologist to an area of potentially active

Figure 5–5. *Duodenal ulcer.*

A, Filled compression views of the duodenal bulb show mild deformity of the cloverleaf type, with a central double density due to pooling in the ulcer (arrow). The outline of a normally shaped bulb is shown on one of the views.

B, Air contrast views. The ulcer is now seen as a collection of barium with a surrounding rim of edema and folds radiating to the collection. Moderate deformity is seen.

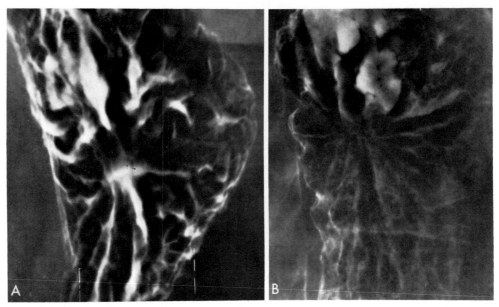

Figure 5–7. *Linear ulcer. A,* A linear ulcer is confirmed when a collection of barium is demonstrated in the center of radiating folds. *B,* If no collection can be demonstrated in the center of the radiating folds, the ulcer has healed, leaving a scar. (From Braver, J. M., et al.: Roentgen diagnosis of linear ulcers. Radiology *132:29,* 1979. Reproduced with permission.)

disease, and a careful search should be made for ulcer craters, particularly linear ones. The double contrast method is valuable for studying these small linear collections, but adequate compression of the bulb using only barium and inherent air will frequently be sufficient to demonstrate a linear ulcer.

Most ulcers heal, some leaving considerable residual scarring as a clue to their past existence; others heal and leave no clues.

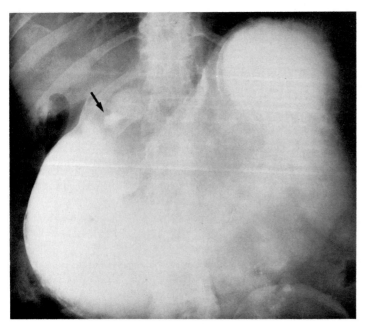

Figure 5–8. *Gastric outlet obstruction* due to a large pyloric channel/base of bulb ulcer. There is massive dilatation of the stomach due to gastric outlet obstruction. A small amount of barium has passed through the pylorus; a pool of contrast material (arrow) in the pyloric canal is an acute ulcer. If gastric outlet obstruction is found, you must try to find the cause; by placing the patient on his right side, enough barium may pass through (or you may be able to manually force enough through) to demonstrate the cause of the obstruction.

Some ulcers have a more complicated course and can be responsible for considerable morbidity and even death. To some extent, the severity of the complication depends on the location of the crater. For example, pyloric channel ulcers frequently cause gastric outlet obstruction because of their location in a vital choke point (Fig. 5–8). Some duodenal ulcers, usually those located on the anterior wall, will perforate into the peritoneal cavity. Posteriorly located ulcers frequently penetrate into the pancreas, causing fulminant pancreatitis, or they may erode into the gastroduodenal artery, resulting in significant hemorrhage. As an aid to memory, recall the saying "anterior perforate, posterior hemorrhage."

POSTBULBAR ULCERS

Postbulbar ulcers probably occur more frequently than realized. They usually are found just distal to the apex of the bulb and on the medial wall of the descending portion of the duodenum (Fig. 5–9). An associated inci-

sura due to spasm can occur on the lateral wall opposite the ulcer. These ulcers are peptic in origin and have the same significance as bulbar ulcers. Postbulbar ulcers characteristically result in significant spasm and deformity, and vomiting is often the predominant symptom. Postbulbar ulcers are frequently difficult to demonstrate but should be suspected with deformity or fold thickening in the postbulbar duodenum.

ZOLLINGER-ELLISON SYNDROME

Multiple ulcers in unusual locations, such as the more distal duodenum or the jejunum, should alert the radiologist to the possibility of the Zollinger-Ellison syndrome. In this disorder, a non–beta islet cell tumor of the pancreas stimulates gastrin production, resulting in excess acid production, which provokes ulcer disease. Usually the stomach contains excess secretions, and the gastric folds are thickened. Ulcerations can occur anywhere, but are typically in the previously mentioned

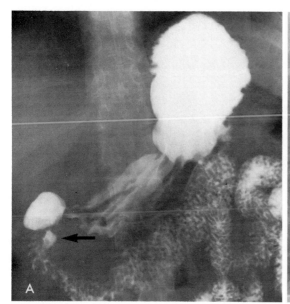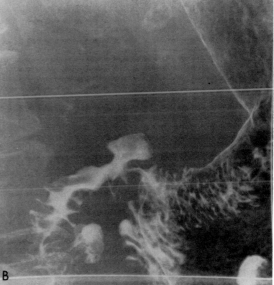

Figure 5–9. *Postbulbar ulcer versus duodenal diverticulum. A,* A collection of barium (arrow) is present on the medial side of the descending limb of the duodenum, with an associated incisura opposite resulting from spasm, and thickening of the neighboring folds. The larger barium pool above the ulcer is in the duodenal bulb which is projecting directly backwards. In *B* a collection of barium is present in the same position in the descending duodenum as in *A,* but this is a diverticulum. Although these are also seen on the inner aspect of the C-sweep, there is no associated spasm or deformity and mucosal folds are seen entering the base of the diverticulum. Incidentally, there is a large ulcer in the duodenal bulb.

"unusual" locations. It should be pointed out, however, that although characteristic, ulcers in unusual sites are not the commonest findings in Zollinger-Ellison syndrome: thickening of the gastric folds associated with thickened folds in the duodenum and jejunum should also suggest this diagnosis. Further radiographic search for the gastrinoma can then be undertaken.

GASTRITIS

This chapter will conclude with a discussion of gastritis, which, although frequently a concomitant of ulcer disease, can occur in other clinical settings. One manifestation of gastritis is thickening of gastric rugae (Fig. 5–10). Normal gastric folds average 4 to 5 mm in width, and folds of this size correlate

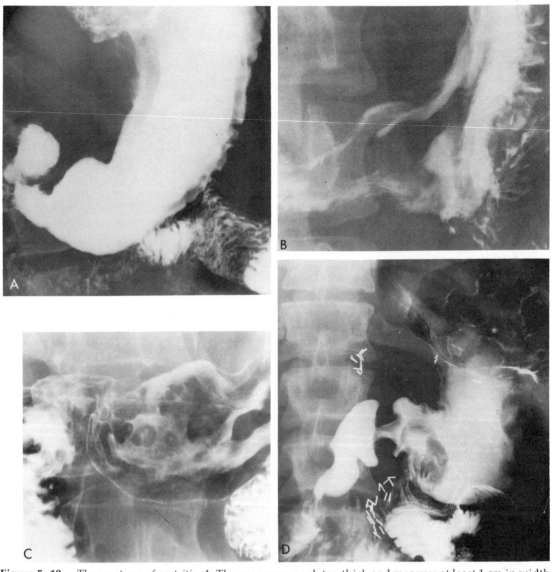

Figure 5–10. *The spectrum of gastritis. A,* The rugae are much too thick and measure at least 1 cm in width. *B,* The folds are even more massive and thickened, measuring 2 cm in width. To the radiologist, these findings indicate gastritis. *C,* Sometimes, actual ulcerations can be demonstrated as collections of barium with a surrounding halo due to edema on the scalloped, thickened folds. *D,* Whenever you see thickened folds, also consider the possibility of lymphoma. In this case, the diagnosis of lymphoma was made with more confidence because there were ulcerated masses distally as well as marked hyperrugosity.

loosely with normal acid output. Normal folds are most obvious on the greater curvature; rugae are usually not seen on the lesser curvature unless they are enlarged. Gastritis due to hyperacidity is probably the most common reason for thickened gastric folds, although other diseases must be considered.

Ménétrier's disease, one of the so-called "protein-losing enteropathies" is characterized by markedly thickened folds in the proximal stomach with antral sparing and hypersecretion. Ingestion of corrosive substances can cause acute edema and thickening of gastric folds. Finally, one must always consider the possibility of tumor infiltration; lymphoma, for example, can present purely as thickened rugae. The absence of a good history for acute gastritis and nonresolution on appropriate medical therapy should alert the radiologist to the possibility of some other etiology.

Basically gastritis is probably not a radiologic diagnosis, and certainly the patient can have a normal upper GI series and still have gastritis. With appropriate history—for example, a recent alcoholic binge—thickened gastric rugae might be interpreted as "gastritis" by the radiologist, but the same finding in the absence of appropriate history might make the diagnosis open to discussion. One type of gastritis, however, can be diagnosed by x-rays with certainty— erosive gastritis. In this entity, the thickened gastric folds become somewhat lumpy and scalloped, and ulcerations with a surrounding rim of edema are seen on these thickened folds. The radiographic appearance of the rounded lucency with a central barium dot is pathognomonic.

For the sake of completeness, it should be mentioned that the folds may also become thinner; this appearance may indicate atrophic gastritis. In gastric atrophy, the folds may be completely absent with a characteristic "bald" fundus. Because gastric atrophy is associated not only with pernicious anemia but also gastric polyps and carcinoma, as much attention should be paid to folds that are too thin as to those that are too thick.

This may seem like a mundane subject, but ulcer disease is "bread and butter" radiology. The general radiologist must be competent in this area to compare favorably with the endoscopist.

References

Stomach (Benign Ulcers)

Bonfield RE, Martel W: The problem of differentiating benign antral ulcers from intramural tumors. Radiology 106:25–27, 1973.

Keller RJ, Wolf BS, Khilnani MT: Roentgen features of healing and healed benign gastric ulcers. Radiology 97:353–359, 1970.

Nelson L: The discovery of gastric ulcers and the differential diagnosis between benignancy and malignancy. Radiol Clin North Am 7:5, 1969.

Wolf BS: Observations of roentgen features of benign and malignant gastric ulcers. Semin Roentgenol 6:140–150, 1971.

Wolf BS, Bryk D: Simple benign prepyloric ulcer. The possibility of an unequivocal roentgen diagnosis. Am J Roentgenol 86:50–60, 1961.

Zboralske FF, Stargardter FL, Harell GS: Profile roentgenographic features of benign greater curvature ulcers. Radiology 127:63–67, 1978.

Stomach (Malignant Ulcers)

Carman RD: Benign and malignant gastric ulcers from a roentgenologic viewpoint. Am J Roentgenol 8:695, 1921.

Carman RD: A new roentgen ray sign of gastric cancer. JAMA 77:990, 1921.

Kirklin BR: The meniscus-complex in the roentgenologic diagnosis of ulcerating carcinoma of the stomach. Am J Roentgenol 47:571, 1942.

Duodenal Ulcers

Sim GPG: The diagnosis of craters in the duodenal cap. Br J Radiol 41:792, 1968.

Stein GN, Martin RD, Roy RH, et al: Evaluation of conventional roentgenographic techniques for demonstration of duodenal ulcer craters. Am J Roentgenol 91:801, 1964.

General

Braver JM, Paul RE Jr, Philipps E, Bloom S: Roentgen diagnosis of linear ulcers. Radiology 132:29, 1979.

Postbulbar Ulcers

Bilbao MK, Frische LH, Rösch J, et al: Postbulbar duodenal ulcer and ring structure. Radiology 100:27, 1971.

Kaufman SA, Levene G: Postbulbar duodenal ulcer. Radiology 69:848, 1957.

Rodriguez HP, Aston JK, Richardson CT: Ulcers in the descending duodenum. Am J Roentgenol 119:316, 1973.

Zollinger-Ellison Syndrome

Amberg JR, Ellison EH, Wilson SD, Zboralske FF: Roentgenographic observations in the Zollinger-Ellison syndrome. JAMA 190:185, 1964.

Nelson SW, Christoforidis AJ: Roentgenologic features of the Zollinger-Ellison Syndrome: ulcerogenic tumor of the pancreas. Semin Roentgenol 3:254, 1968.

Gastritis

Chokas WV, Conner DH: Giant hypertrophy of gastric mucosa, hypoproteinemia and edema (Ménétrier's disease). Am J Med 27:125, 1959.

Poplack W, Paul RE, Goldsmith M, Matsue H, Moore JP, Norton R: Demonstration of erosive gastritis by the double-contrast technique. Radiology 117:519–521, 1975.

6

"INFLAMMATORY" DISEASE (THE "-ITISES")

Under this broad umbrella an overview of how inflammation may affect the GI tract will be given. Again the principles will be stressed; inflammation, wherever it occurs, has a very similar radiographic appearance, and the student can learn to recognize an inflammatory process anywhere in the GI tract.

The radiographic appearance of an inflammatory process will vary depending on where in the wall it is located and whether the layer predominantly involved is the mucosa, the submucosa (submucosal lesions are also known as intramural), or the serosa.

MUCOSAL INFLAMMATION

The hallmark of *mucosal* inflammation is *ulceration*. If the ulceration is extremely shallow, the only radiographic finding may be granularity of the mucosa or a shaggy or spiculated edge to the barium; if deeper, actual erosions or ulcers will be seen. If seen en face, an ulcer will appear as a collection of barium; if profiled, it will look like a projection; if empty, it will be a ring. Any elevated edema mound will displace the barium and therefore will be seen as a translucent halo surrounding the central collection. *Spasm* or irritability with resultant deformity is com-

monly associated with an inflammatory process, as is a localized ileus. The bowel lumen may be narrowed by the edema or spasm, but the mucosa (apart from the ulcer itself) is intact; this distinguishes spasm from infiltration due to a malignant process. On healing, the ulcerated area may return completely to normal, may scar and result in radiating folds, or may fibrose, resulting in either shortening of the bowel or narrowing of the lumen. This is how a benign stricture develops after esophagitis or how the lesser curvature shortens following a lesser curvature ulcer. In extreme form, when ulcerative colitis heals, the result is a short colon with no haustra, the so-called "lead-pipe" colon.

Acute mucosal inflammation may have many causes; among the precipitating factors are *infections* (e.g., Candida or herpes in the esophagus); *toxins* (in the broad sense of the word, to include the irritative effect of gastric acid on the esophageal mucosa or of bile on the stomach); and *exogenous irritants*, such as alcohol, aspirin, lye, and many other drugs given orally. Radiation may also result in mucosal inflammation. Often the cause of the inflammation is unknown, in which case it is termed *idiopathic*.

In general, as we have said, the infectious and "toxic" group produce mucosal inflammation with ulceration, edema, and associated spasm; apart from the target organ and the amount of spasm, the appearance is very similar. Occasionally a distinguishing feature of Candida esophagitis can be the formation of linear deeper ulcers, and there are often associated filling defects due to the fungal plaques. Sometimes the location of the inflammatory process will give a clue to the underlying cause — e.g., lye esophagitis is most marked at normal areas where the barium holds up, such as the aortic arch.

SUBMUCOSAL INFLAMMATION

If the inflammation is deeper, so that the *submucosa* is involved (for example, in Crohn's disease), not only will the ulcers be deeper, but also the bowel wall will become thickened. Normally, the loops of bowel fit closely together; when an abnormal loop is widely separated from adjacent loops, one can assume that the wall of that loop is thick.

Many things can cause thickening of the wall: blood, edema fluid, or actual tissue infiltration. In submucosal inflammation, the folds become thicker and are seen as more obvious bands crossing the bowel lumen. Similarly, the bowel contour may become scalloped by soft tissue masses indenting the lumen; how big the scallops are depends on which part of the bowel is involved. Thus, "thumbprinting" is the hallmark of submucosal fluid in the colon, whereas "pinky-printing" indicates submucosal fluid in the small bowel. This appearance merely means that there is excess fluid or tissue in the submucosa; radiologically, edema and blood are indistinguishable, and the clinical history and related findings will help to clarify the etiology.

SEROSAL INFLAMMATION

Inflammation may also involve the *serosa*, either from within or from an adjacent extrinsic inflammatory process, e.g., peridiverticulitis, endometriosis. The serosa will then be tugged into small projections known as spiculations, and the inflammatory mass may indent or displace the bowel. Eventually, serosal inflammation may cause scars resulting in adhesions, the most common cause of small bowel obstruction. The involved loops will be tethered and sharply angulated.

There is, however, one real problem with serosal disease. Unlike *mucosal* diseases, in which it is usually possible to distinguish between inflammation (when the folds will be thick but intact) and infiltration (when the folds will be distorted or destroyed), with pure *serosal* disease usually this distinction is not possible. For example, radiographically endometriosis may look exactly like serosal metastases. In most cases, it is possible to say that serosal disease is present, but not whether it is inflammatory or metastatic. Other clinical parameters will clarify this dilemma.

RADIOGRAPHIC APPEARANCE OF INFLAMMATORY PROCESSES

So, many organs may become inflamed, resulting in a combination of the above findings, depending on whether the mucosa, submucosa, or serosa bears the brunt of the insult. Thus, esophagitis, regardless of whether it is due to reflux of acid, infection, or exogenous toxin, will result in spasm and irritability; ulcers will be seen as shagginess or erosions; the esophageal folds will be thickened and edematous. Similarly, gastritis may manifest itself as thickened folds alone, or actual erosions may be seen. Other inflammatory diseases will be manifested primarily as serosal inflammation. Thus, diverticulitis due to perforation of a diverticulum, or endometriosis due to *serosal* implants, will result in spiculation, tethering, and mass effect. Similarly, appendicitis may result in mass effect on the cecum and serosal inflammation.

Inflammatory processes often result in a reflex ileus in nearby bowel; thus, a "sentinel loop" may be seen in the midabdomen in pancreatitis or in the right lower quadrant in appendicitis. There are actually two common ileus patterns in pancreatitis: a dilated loop of duodenum or jejunum, or dilatation and apparent abrupt termination of the transverse

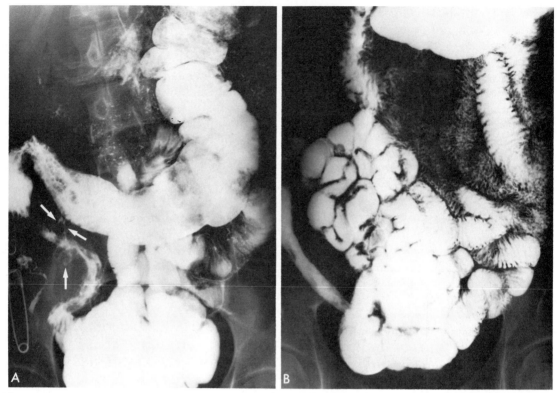

Figure 6–1. *A, Crohn's disease of terminal ileum and right colon.* The terminal ileum is nodular, with a very thick wall, and the right colon is short and ahaustral. There are multiple fistulae (arrows) between the terminal ileum and right colon. Incidentally, this patient presented with a psoas abscess due to another fistula from the diseased bowel to the psoas muscle.

B, Crohn's disease. There is a markedly abnormal small bowel loop in the right lower quadrant with luminal narrowing, multiple nodular filling defects, and marked thickening of the bowel wall, as evidenced by the displacement of the abnormal loop from its nearby normal neighbors. The remainder of the small bowel follow-through appears normal.

colon, the so-called "colon cut-off" sign. In appendicitis, the ileus will involve a few loops of distal small bowel.

Following this brief discussion of inflammatory processes in general, the two major idiopathic inflammatory bowel diseases of Western society, namely, *Crohn's disease* and *ulcerative colitis* will be described.

CROHN'S DISEASE

Inflammatory bowel disease that involves the small bowel alone (Crohn's disease, regional enteritis) usually presents little diagnostic problem, although it may sometimes be difficult to distinguish between Crohn's disease and lymphoma. A small bowel follow-through is essential in the search for abnormal loops, and special attention should be paid to the terminal ileum, a favored site (Fig. 6–1). Other areas of the small bowel, however, may be involved. Look for ulcers, spiculation and nodulation; the lumen will be narrowed and the wall markedly thickened. Spasm produces even more luminal narrowing, resulting eventually in the "string sign." Classically, if more than one area of small bowel is involved, abnormal segments alternate with normal bowel, resulting in "skip" lesions (Fig. 6–2). As well as the small bowel, Crohn's disease can occur anywhere in the GI tract, from mouth to anus. Involvement of the stomach and duodenum is becoming increasingly recognized (Fig. 6–3), especially with air contrast studies; esophageal involvement is less common.

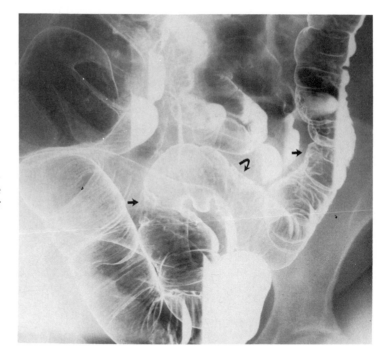

Figure 6–2. *Crohn's disease of the colon with multiple "skip" areas* (arrows). Note that the abnormal areas are asymmetric and eccentric, and consist both of surface irregularity and projecting linear ulcerations (curved arrow).

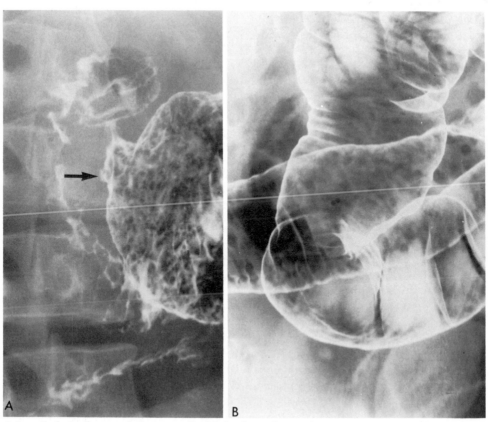

Figure 6–3. *Crohn's disease of the stomach.* Multiple apthous ulcers are present in the antrum, plus a deeper ulcer (arrow) on the greater curvature distally. Notice how the distal antrum does not distend completely, confirming inflammation. The duodenal C-sweep is markedly contracted, with swollen, edematous folds; other films showed that the duodenum also was involved by skip lesions. *B,* Aphthous ulcers in the colon are identical to the lesions in *A.*

It is when the colon is involved that a problem arises — how to differentiate between *granulomatous colitis* (Crohn's colitis), and *ulcerative colitis* (UC). Until fairly recently (early 1960's) this was not a problem at all, as it was not known that Crohn's disease could involve the colon. Indeed, it may be that many or all of those patients previously described as having "segmental ulcerative colitis" in fact had Crohn's disease.

Exactly why is it so important to make this distinction? How does it affect the patient?

DISTINGUISHING BETWEEN CROHN'S DISEASE AND ULCERATIVE COLITIS

The prognosis, treatment, and potential complications of these two diseases differ widely. It is important, therefore, to be able to differentiate between the two with some degree of confidence, so that appropriate therapy and follow-up can be instituted. Radiology plays a major role both in confirming the diagnosis and in assessing the extent, severity, and activity of the disease. X-ray study is also vital to look for any complications, e.g., carcinoma in ulcerative colitis, fistulae or abscesses in Crohn's disease. Radiology and endoscopy should be thought of not as competitive but as complementary procedures in the management of these diseases.

The incidence of carcinoma is markedly increased in long-standing UC; in pancolitis, the risk increases the younger the age of onset and the longer the duration of disease. Radiology, supplemented by endoscopy, plays an important role in its detection (Fig. 6–4). Any stricture should be viewed with alarm, even if it appears benign. Carcinoma in this disease tends to be plaque-like and not polypoidal, but any suspicious area should be biopsied to exclude carcinoma. Recently, the x-ray findings of a precancerous change in the mucosa, intestinal dysplasia, were described and areas showing such changes should also be biopsied. Incidentally, it is now agreed that there is also a higher incidence of carcinoma in patients with long-standing Crohn's disease.

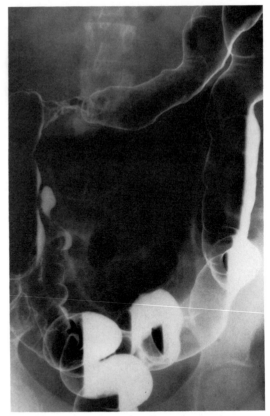

Figure 6–4. *Carcinoma in ulcerative colitis.* The risk of developing carcinoma for patients with long-standing pancolitis is markedly increased over that for the general population. Few of these are of the polypoid type, so any stricture in these patients must be considered cancer until proved otherwise. This is amply illustrated by this patient; the stricture in the hepatic flexure was carcinoma.

If surgery is performed in UC, e.g., for toxic dilatation or intractable bloody diarrhea, a colectomy and ileostomy is curvative. Crohn's disease, however, is a recurrent disease and, even if severe strictures and fistulae necessitate surgery, the disease often will recur, most often at the anastomosis.

RADIOGRAPHIC DISTINCTION BETWEEN ULCERATIVE COLITIS AND GRANULOMATOUS COLITIS

If, therefore, the radiologist is faced with an ulcerating disease that involves the colon and if one of the "idiopathic" inflammatory bowel diseases is present and not some un-

TABLE 6–1. ULCERATIVE VERSUS GRANULOMATOUS COLITIS

	Ulcerative	Granulomatous
General Features	Continuous Symmetrical Concentric	Discontinuous ("skip" areas) Asymmetrical Eccentric
Rectum	Involved in 96%	Not involved in 50%
Anus	Normal	Diseased—perianal fissures and fistulae
Terminal ileum	Dilated and patulous ("backwash ileitis")	Narrowed and inflamed ("string sign")
Ulcers	A mucosal disease— ulcers are superficial	A submucosal disease— ulcers are deep
Fistula formation	No—rare	Yes—common
Pseudopolyps	Common (20%)	Yes but per cent unknown
Cancer potential	Markedly increased with total colitis and in- creasing duration of disease	Still being evaluated but increased in small bowel, thought to be increased in colon
Toxic dilatation	1% will present this way	Yes, but less common

common infectious process such as Salmonella infection or amebic dysentery, how can ulcerative colitis and granulomatous colitis be differentiated? Sometimes this is easy and sometimes it is very difficult, but attention to certain points will clarify in most cases (Table 6–1).

Ask the following questions:

1. How is the colon affected? Are continuous or skip lesions present? Are lesions concentric or eccentric? Symmetrical or asymmetrical?

2. Is there small bowel involvement? What does the terminal ileum look like?

3. Is there rectal disease? Anal or perianal disease?

4. Are there fistulae?

The radiologist should then decide whether the disease is active or burnt-out; chronic colitis results in the shortened ahaustral colon familiar to all, but the presence of *ulcers* means active disease, which requires more intensive therapy.

ULCERS. The ulcers in these two diseases differ. In ulcerative colitis, the whole mucosa is abnormal, with a spectrum of findings from the fine granularity of mucosal edema, to a coarsely granular appearance, to deeper ulcers (Fig. 6–5); this was demonstrated with beautiful endoscopic correlation in the classic paper by Laufer and colleagues. In Crohn's disease the hallmark is the "aphthous" ulcer (similar in appearance to aphthoid mouth ulcers); these are discrete ulcers surrounded by an edema mound on a background of *normal mucosa*. Like the nodules of miliary tuberculosis, these ulcers can be "picked up with a pair of forceps." Aphthous ulcers due to Crohn's disease may also be demonstrated elsewhere (e.g., stomach, duodenum) if air contrast techniques are used. Note the similarity of these ulcers to erosions elsewhere in the gut!

It used to be said that the shape of the ulcers themselves was also different. The "collar-button" ulcer was said to be characteristic of UC, the "rose-thorn" type of granulomatous colitis. This is no longer thought to be the case; the *depth* of the ulcer rather than the shape is more important (shallow in ulcerative colitis and deep in Crohn's disease). The deep linear ulcers of Crohn's disease may form an intersecting network, resulting in a characteristic appearance called cobblestoning

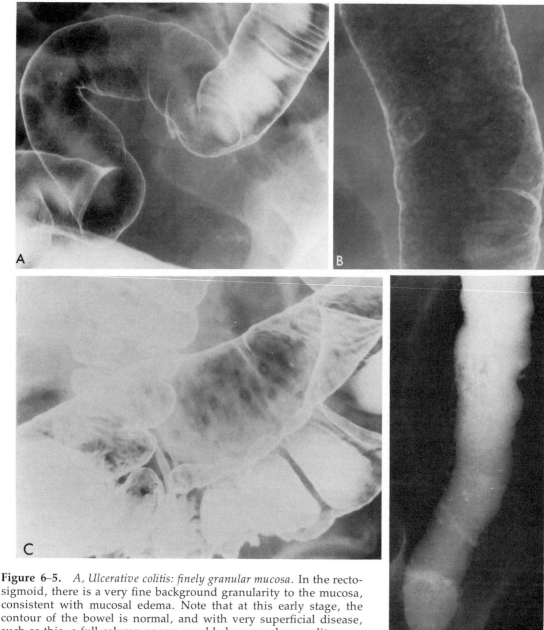

Figure 6–5. *A, Ulcerative colitis: finely granular mucosa.* In the rectosigmoid, there is a very fine background granularity to the mucosa,
consistent with mucosal edema. Note that at this early stage, the
contour of the bowel is normal, and with very superficial disease,
such as this, a full-column enema would show no abnormality.

B, Ulcerative colitis: coarsely granular appearance. The normal fea-
tureless background pattern of the colon has been replaced by a very coarse granular appearance due to
barium trapped in multiple shallow ulcerations. The contour of the bowel is still probably normal.
Incidentally, the circle in the center of the picture represents coating of an isolated pseudopolyp.

C, Crohn's disease: aphthous ulcers. Multiple rounded filling defects with a central ulcer crater indicate the
aphthous ulcers of Crohn's disease. Note that these ulcers are discrete and the intervening mucosa is
completely normal.

D, Collar-button ulcers. Multiple collections of barium representing ulcers are seen en face and in profile
in the descending colon of this full-column enema. These flask-shaped ulcers are known as collar-button
ulcers. It was thought that these were specific for ulcerative colitis, but they can be seen in the other
ulcerating colitides. This particular patient had *Salmonella typhi* infection.

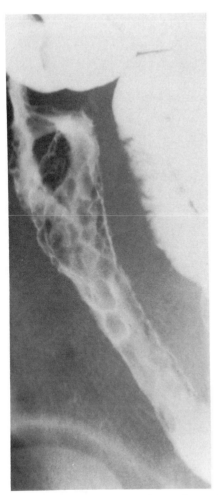

Figure 6–6. *Cobblestoning* (Crohn's disease). A coned-down view of the terminal ileum shows nodular filling defects combined with intersecting barium collections. This is due to a network of intersecting linear ulcers and is called cobblestoning. Supporting evidence for Crohn's disease is the double lumen distally, indicating fistulization, and the increase in wall thickness.

(Fig. 6–6) — a term which has been much misused and abused.

PSEUDOPOLYPS. As the ulcers heal, any remaining normal mucosa becomes hyperplastic, resulting in tissue mounds, the so-called "pseudopolyps" (Fig. 6–7) (perhaps a better term is "postinflammatory polyps"). These may occur in either disease and merely mean there has been severe mucosal disease in the past. Occasionally these frondlike polyps may become very large and may even

cause obstruction. An unusual type of pseudopolyp is the threadlike filiform polyp or mucosal bridge.

With healing, the colon may return completely to normal or may lose its haustra and shorten, resulting in the "lead-pipe" colon, a sign of "burnt-out" colitis. Long-term laxative abuse can be confused with chronic UC; unlike UC, however, the changes are more prominent in the right colon and, although ahaustral, the colon is not shortened.

Two other areas are important in deciding which disease is present; these are the *rectum* and the *terminal ileum.*

RECTAL DISEASE. The rectal mucosa is assessed for ulceration or lack of distensibility (Fig. 6–8). If a full-column study is performed, the rectum may appear normal and still be diseased; attention should then be directed to the presacral space, which is normally less than 1.5 cm (in obese people it may be as much as 2 cm). With rectal involvement, this space will be widened owing to perirectal inflammation, and the rectum will appear tubular. The rectum is diseased in almost all patients with UC, but is spared in at least 50 per cent of patients with Crohn's disease. *Anal* disease, on the other hand, is highly specific for Crohn's disease and it is marked by perianal fissures and fistulae.

ILEAL DISEASE. The appearance of the terminal ileum is also important. Ulcerative colitis is a colonic disease affecting the terminal ileum secondarily. "Backwash ileitis" may be seen in pancolitis; the terminal ileum is patulous and dilated, with a wide-open ileocecal valve. Crohn's disease, on the other hand, may affect any site in the gastrointestinal tract, although the favorite spot is the terminal ileum. The terminal ileum will become nodular, ulcerated, inflamed, and thick-walled; fistulae may or may not be present.

Unlike the situation with the colon, where ulcers will be seen when disease is active, it is often extremely difficult to assess the activity of small bowel Crohn's disease by x-ray. This merely reflects the known inaccuracy of the small bowel follow-through; ulceration may not be demonstrated unless enteroclysis is performed.

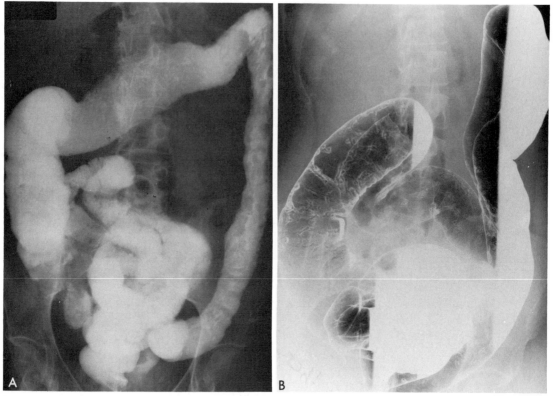

Figure 6–7. *A, Ulcerative colitis with pseudopolyps.* A full-column enema shows a shortened ahaustral colon with multiple filling defects in the descending colon. These filling defects are mounds of hyperplastic tissue known as pseudopolyps.

B, Filiform pseudopolyps. An air contrast barium enema shows a somewhat ahaustral but certainly not shortened colon. There are multiple linear filamentous filling defects representing unusually shaped pseudopolyps known as filiform polyps.

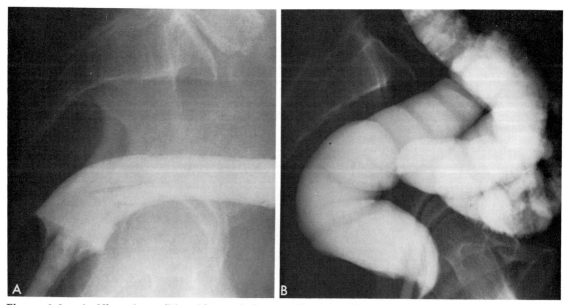

Figure 6–8. *A, Ulcerative colitis with rectal disease.* On this full-column enema, the rectum appears indistensible and tubular. There is widening of the presacral space due to perirectal inflammation. Note that the rectal balloon has been partially inflated, which is, in fact, contraindicated in patients with inflammatory bowel disease. *B, Normal lateral film of the rectum,* for comparison.

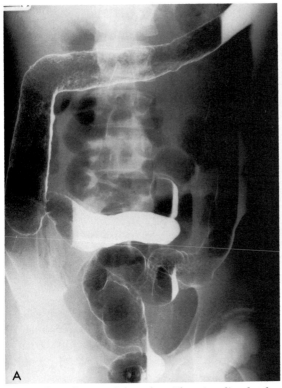
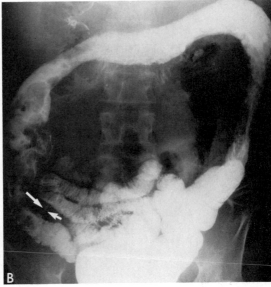

Figure 6–9. *A, Total ulcerative colitis with backwash ileitis.* The whole colon is involved and appears short and ahaustral, with a coarsely granular mucosal pattern. The terminal ileum is dilated and patulous, consistent with "backwash ileitis." Note also the narrowed area in the midrectum, raising the question of a carcinoma.

B, Crohn's disease of the colon. The visualized colon is short and ahaustral, with multiple nodular filling defects consistent with pseudopolyps; other films showed the rectum was spared. The wall of the terminal ileum is thickened, and there is a fistula from the terminal ileum to the adjacent loop of small bowel. In addition, the duodenum is outlined by contrast medium via a fistula from the hepatic flexure.

Once the radiologist knows *what* to look for, how is the study chosen that will produce the highest diagnostic yield?

TOXIC DILATATION (TOXIC MEGACOLON)

First of all, a word of caution. The barium enema, indeed any enema and even bowel preparation, has been implicated in the subsequent development of toxic dilatation. Is a barium enema really potentially dangerous in the patient with inflammatory bowel disease? Just what is "toxic dilatation?"

To answer the second question first, "toxic dilatation" (toxic megacolon) is a medical emergency in which a patient with inflammatory bowel disease presents with fever, severe bloody diarrhea, and a *distended colon* (Fig. 6–10). One in 100 patients with UC will present in this way; fewer but a still significant number of patients, with Crohn's disease

will develop this complication. Toxic dilatation has also been reported in amebic dysentery and ischemic colitis.

"Toxicity" is a clinical diagnosis; the dilatation, however, is visible on x-rays. Certain measurements have been worked out for the normal colon: cecum, < 9 cm; transverse colon, < 6 cm. Measurements greater than these mean the colon is dilated and there is an increased risk of perforation. This risk is, of course, greater for a given degree of distention if the colon also happens to be diseased. In toxic megacolon, a colon with severe mucosal disease is also becoming increasingly distended. What causes this dilatation is not known; it is a kind of reflex ileus.

As with any dilated bowel, the decision must be made whether the bowel is dilated but otherwise normal or dilated and diseased — e.g., inflamed or ischemic. In some cases there may be signs of chronic inflammatory bowel disease to provide clues, such as

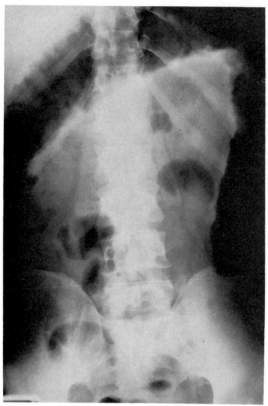

Figure 6–10. *Toxic dilatation.* The colon is not only markedly dilated but also short and ahaustral; there are multiple soft tissue densities, pseudopolyps, and wall edema.

loss of haustration and soft tissue mounds (pseudopolyps). Signs of acute inflammation might also be present, such as submucosal edema (thumb-printing).

The radiologist must immediately signal these danger signs of mucosal disease and dilatation to the clinician. Intensive resuscitative measures must be instituted (high-dose steroids, intravenous fluids, antibiotics) and the patient followed carefully both by clinical examination and with plain abdominal films. A danger sign is increasing bowel distention despite intensive treatment; of course, the dreaded complication of toxic megacolon is *perforation.*

OBSTRUCTION VERSUS INFLAMMATORY DISEASE

It is most important to be able to differentiate between dilatation due to obstruction and dilatation due to acute inflammatory disease. To diagnose obstruction, barium enema is needed, whereas a barium enema is *absolutely contraindicated* in the patient with toxic megacolon. *This patient should not have an enema under any circumstances.* This point cannot be stressed too much; patients with *acute* inflammatory bowel disease who have any evidence of megacolon on an abdominal film should have *no study at all;* the gastroenterologist will show the same caution and will not perform colonoscopy. The increase in intraluminal pressure from the enema may be enough to perforate the colon; even insertion of the enema tip may perforate the diseased rectal mucosa. See Table 6–2 for guidelines for performing examinations in inflammatory bowel disease.

What about patients with acute bloody diarrhea and suspected inflammatory bowel disease who have no signs of toxic megacolon? Often the patient with severe bloody diarrhea will not require either an oral bowel preparation or a cleanout enema. In fact, many clinicians are unwilling to prepare the acute patient; both oral cathartics and washout enemas have been known to exacerbate acute inflammatory bowel disease. Fortunately, it turns out that preparation more stringent than a "liquids only" diet often is not necessary in the *acute* phase because solid stool theoretically will not adhere to inflamed mucosa. This is the basis for the "instant enema" in the patient with ulcerative colitis. Barium is run in gently until it hits solid stool; at this point or close to it the colon presumably is normal. This technique will usually underestimate the extent of the disease process.

If the patient's disease is quiescent or if he has relatively mild symptoms, it is safe to

TABLE 6–2. IMPORTANT POINTS TO REMEMBER IN RADIOGRAPHY OF INFLAMMATORY BOWEL DISEASE

Scout KUB film extremely important in assessing for colonic dilatation and colon cleansing.
Tailor examination to clinical question.
Insert enema tip with care.
Do not inflate rectal balloon.
Do not overdistend the bowel.
Use speed.

go ahead and give a *gentle* cleansing enema followed by a *gentle, speedy* contrast enema. In general, if the clinician is willing to prepare the patient, the radiologist should be able to perform a gentle washout enema. The colon should be as clean as possible to obviate confusion between stool and pseudopolyps, especially the unusually shaped filiform pseudopolyps.

CHOICE OF ENEMA

The question to be asked now is: what sort of enema should be performed, air contrast or full-column? How much is revealed on radiography depends on which technique is used. A full-column enema will show deep ulcers, whereas shallow ulcers and mucosal edema may be seen only when air contrast is used. In fact, because the full-column technique will not show superficial mucosal disease, it is possible to have a "normal" single contrast study and the patient still have significant inflammatory bowel disease.

Is this important or not? We believe it is, for two important reasons: accurate diagnosis and appropriate follow-up. It is essential for successful follow-up to know how extensive the disease is; there is a markedly increased risk of developing carcinoma in patients with pancolitis. In these patients, follow-up studies are directed at finding this carcinoma and, if the disease extent has been underestimated — or, even worse, the diagnosis not even made, the necessary follow-up will not be carried out. The authors have seen two patients in whom a full-column enema was completely normal; these patients had no follow-up studies and returned between 5 and 10 years later not only with full-blown chronic inflammatory bowel disease but, more importantly, also with advanced carcinoma. We would therefore recommend that air contrast be performed, both for suspected cases of inflammatory bowel disease and in follow-up studies of known cases.

Basically then, the choice of study depends on the *clinical situation* and the *status of the disease process.* Is the patient an ambulatory patient with some bloody diarrhea that is not incapacitating, or is the disease process relatively quiescent? Is this a "rule-out inflammatory bowel disease" or are we looking for *complications* of known disease? Many factors should be taken into consideration in deciding which enema, if any, to perform.

Sometimes radiologists find themselves in a real quandary about which study to perform. An example might be trying to exclude Crohn's disease when the terminal ileum has not been seen on a routine small bowel examination. A single contrast study with reflux into the terminal ileum would solve this problem, but early disease in the colon may be missed unless an air contrast colon study is performed.

Whatever study is chosen, it should be done quickly, avoiding overdistention of the colon. It is extremely important not to inflate the rectal balloon (a rule in anyone suspected of having a diseased rectum). The tip should be inserted with great care, because of the risk of pushing the tip straight through the friable mucosa. As these patients usually have severe spasm and tenesmus, an antispasmodic (glucagon) can be extremely helpful and should be used whenever possible.

OTHER ENTEROCOLITIDES

Pseudomembranous Colitis ("Toxin-induced" or Antibiotic-Related Colitis)

An increasing number of patients with this disease entity are being seen, and it has now been described with almost every antibiotic used and even without antibiotic use. Characteristically there is a positive titer to the toxin of *Clostridium difficile.* Dramatic response follows treatment with vancomycin.

Characteristic findings have been described on both plain films and contrast studies (Fig. 6–11). On the plain film, broad bands of soft tissue crossing the colon are characteristic although not always seen; the findings may be less specific and mimic ulcerative or ischemic colitis. If a contrast study is performed, the plaques (pseudomembranes) will be seen as filling defects within the barium column; this is in contrast to the ulcers seen in the ulcerating colitides.

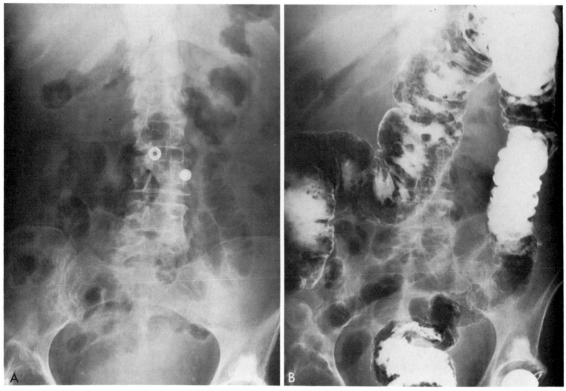

Figure 6–11. *Pseudomembranous Colitis*

A, Plain film findings in pseudomembranous colitis. This plain film demonstrates broad transverse bands of soft tissue within the gas shadow of the transverse colon, which are too thick to be confused with normal haustra. Transverse bands or thumb-prints should suggest pseudomembranous colitis, although thumb-printing by itself, in the appropriate clinical setting, would also raise the question of ischemia.

B, On barium enema, the colon length and haustration appear normal. There are multiple filling defects representing the plaques or pseudomembranes. (By courtesy of H. F. Gramm, New England Deaconess Hospital, Boston, Massachusetts.)

UNUSUAL CAUSES OF COLITIS IN OUR SOCIETY

Tuberculosis

Tuberculosis of the terminal ileum and colon is extremely uncommon in Western cultures, whereas it is rampant in the Far East. One should mention tuberculosis in the same breath as Crohn's disease just to dismiss it. The findings in this condition may be identical with those of Crohn's disease.

Amebic Colitis

Another unusual cause of colitis in our society is amebic infection. The colitis may be segmental (cecum or rectum most commonly) or involve the whole colon. The same findings of ulceration and inflammation are present, but characteristically the terminal ileum is spared, an important distinguishing feature from Crohn's disease or tuberculosis.

MISCELLANEOUS

Other infections, such as with Salmonella, may give a picture identical to UC. The uncommon Behçet's syndrome may mimic UC. Remember also that ischemic colitis may eventually ulcerate, producing an "ulcerating" colitis. Yersinia ileitis and Campylobacter infection can simulate Crohn's disease.

To all intents and purposes, however,

when one encounters an ulcerating or inflammatory bowel disease in everyday practice, the differential diagnosis is between ulcerative colitis and granulomatous disease.

References

General

Brodey PA, Hill RP, Baron S: Benign ulceration of the cecum. Radiology 122:323–327, 1977.

Hammerman AM, Shatz BA, Susman N: Radiographic characteristics of colonic "mucosal bridges:" sequelae of inflammatory bowel disease. Radiology 127:611, 1978.

Zegel HG, Laufer I: Filiform polyposis. Radiology 127:615, 1978.

Crohn's Disease

Ekberg O, Fork FT, Hildell J: Predictive value of small bowel radiography for recurrent Crohn's disease. Am J Roentgenol 135:1051–1055, 1980.

Joffe N, Antonioli DA, Bettmann MA, Goldman H: Focal granulomatous (Crohn's) colitis: radiologic-pathologic correlation. Gastrointest Radioi 3:73–80, 1978.

Laufer I, Costopoulos L: Early lesions of Crohn's disease. Am J Roentgenol 130:307–311, 1978.

Lightdale CJ, Sternberg SS, Posner G, Sherlock P: Carcinoma complicating Crohn's disease. Report of seven cases and review of the literature. Am J Med 59:262–268, 1975.

Marshak RH: Granulomatous disease of the intestinal tract (Crohn's disease). Annual Oration in Honor of Benjamin H. Ordnoff, M.D., 1881–1971. Radiology 114:3, 1975.

Simpkins KC: Some aspects of the radiology of Crohn's disease. Br J Surg 59:810–817, 1972.

Differentiation Between Ulcerative Colitis and Granulomatous Colitis

Kelvin FM, Oddson TA, Rice RP, Garbutt JT, Bradenham BP: Double contrast barium enema in Crohn's disease and ulcerative colitis. Am J Roentgenol 131:207, 1978.

Laufer I: Air contrast studies of the colon in inflammatory bowel disease. Crit Rev Radiol 9:421, 1977.

Laufer I, Mullens JE, Hamilton J: Correlation of endoscopy and double-contrast radiography in the early stages of ulcerative and granulomatous colitis. Radiology 118:1–5, 1976.

Margulis AR, Goldberg HI, Lawson TL, Montgomery CK, Rambo ON, Noonan CD, Amberg JR: The overlapping spectrum of ulcerative and granulomatous colitis: a roentgenographic-pathologic study. Am J Roentgenol 113:325, 1971.

Stanley P, Kelsey FI, Dawson AM, Dyer N: Radiological signs of ulcerative colitis and Crohn's disease of the colon. Clin Radiol 22:434–442, 1971.

Thoeni RF, Margulis AR: Radiology in inflammatory diseases of the colon: an area of increased interest for the modern clinician. Invest Radiol 15:281–292, 1980.

Ulcerative Colitis

Bartram CI: Radiology in the current assessment of ulcerative colitis. Gastrointest Radiol 1:383–392, 1977.

Bartram CI, Walmsley K: A radiological and pathological correlation of the mucosal changes in ulcerative colitis. Clin Radiol 29:323, 1978.

Binder SC, Patterson JF, Glotzer DJ: Toxic megacolon in ulcerative colitis. Gastroenterology 66:909–915, 1974.

Fennessy JJ, Sparberg MB, Kirsner JB: Radiological findings in carcinoma of the colon complicating chronic ulcerative colitis. Gut 9:388–397, 1968.

Frank PH, Riddell RH, Feczko PJ, Levin B: Radiological detection of colonic dysplasia (precarcinoma) in chronic ulcerative colitis. Gastrointest Radiol 3:209–220, 1978.

Hinton JM: Risk of malignant change in ulcerative colitis. Gut 7:427–432, 1966.

Hodgson JR, Sauer WG: The roentgenologic features of carcinoma in chronic ulcerative colitis. Am J Roentgenol 86:91–96, 1961.

Jones JH, Chapman M: Definition of megacolon in colitis. Gut 10:562–564, 1969.

Lichtenstein JE, Madewell JE, Feigin DS: The collar button ulcer. A radiologic-pathologic correlation. Gastrointest Radiol 4:79–84, 1979.

Other Inflammatory Diseases

Balikian JP, Uthman SM, Khouri NF: Intestinal amebiasis: a roentgen analysis of 19 cases including two case reports. Am J Roentgenol 122:245, 1974.

Carrera GF, Young S, Lewicki AM: Intestinal tuberculosis. Gastrointest Radiol 1:147–155, 1976.

Kolawole TM, Lewis EA: Radiologic observations on intestinal amebiasis. Am J Roentgenol 122:257, 1974.

Kolawole TM, Lewis EA: A radiologic study of tuberculosis of the abdomen (gastrointestinal tract). Am J Roentgenol 123:348, 1975.

Thoeni RF, Margulis AR: Gastrointestinal tuberculosis. Semin Roentgenol 14:283, 1979.

Pseudomembranous Colitis

Stanley RJ, Melson GL, Tedesco FJ: The spectrum of radiographic findings in antibiotic-related pseudomembranous colitis. Radiology 111:519–524, 1974.

Stanley RJ, Melson GL, Tedesco FJ, Saylor JL: Plain-film findings in severe pseudomembranous colitis. Radiology 118:7–11, 1976.

Herpes Zoster

Menuck LS, Brahme F, Amberg J, Sherr HP: Colonic changes of herpes zoster. Am J Roentgenol 127:273, 1976.

Yersinia Infections

Ekberg O, Sjostrom B, Brahme F: Radiological findings in Yersinia ileitis. Radiology 123:15–19, 1977.

Lachman R, Soong J, Wishon G, Maenza R, Hanelin L, St Geme J: Yersinia colitis. Gastrointest Radiol 2:133–135, 1977.

7
NEOPLASM

Cancer is the second leading cause of death in the United States. Cancer of the digestive tract, notably the colon and rectum, is second only to lung cancer in men, and breast and lung cancer in women, as the cause of cancer deaths. In the over 75 population, digestive tract cancer is the leading cause of death.

Although all tumors certainly are not malignant, the importance of detecting those that *may* be cannot be overestimated. This is especially true in certain high-risk groups prone to the development of GI tract malignancy (Table 7–1).

TABLE 7–1.   HIGH-RISK FACTORS FOR GI TRACT MALIGNANCY

Esophagus
  Smoking, alcohol, other food carcinogens
  Sideropenic dysphagia (Plummer-Vinson syndrome)
  Achalasia
  Columnar epithelium–lined esophagus
  Lye ingestion
Stomach
  Gastric atrophy
  Adenomatous polyps in pernicious anemia
  Post gastrectomy
  Asbestosis
Small Bowel
  Crohn's disease
  Sprue
Colon
  Familial polyposis
  Gardner's syndrome
  Ulcerative colitis
  Granulomatous colitis
  Ureterosigmoidostomy

DIAGNOSING MALIGNANCY

The GI radiologist plays a critical role in detecting neoplastic disease and in assessing its impact on patient survival. It is his job to *find the lesion.* Once a lesion has been found, there are a number of questions to be answered:

1. Is the lesion *benign* or *malignant*? That is, does it have *smooth, tapering* edges (Fig. 7–1) with *normal peristalsis* and *intact mucosa* (benign) or does it have *overhanging, shouldered* borders and *absent peristalsis*, rigidity, and *destroyed mucosa* (malignant)?

By what means can the mucosa be judged to be intact? Look carefully at the fold pattern; the small bowel folds and colon haustra must be present, and neither distorted nor destroyed. The postevacuation film of a single column study can be particularly helpful here as there is a definite feathery appearance to the normal contracted colon (Fig. 7–2). A destructive mucosal lesion may become more obvious on the postevacuation film because it cannot contract normally.

2. Is the lesion *solitary* or *multiple*? It is especially important to look for a second colonic cancer; some 4 to 5 per cent of these cancers are concurrent.

3. Is the lesion *confined to the bowel* or are there signs of *spread*, either locally or distantly?

When the radiologist identifies a lesion, he should attempt to classify it as either (a)

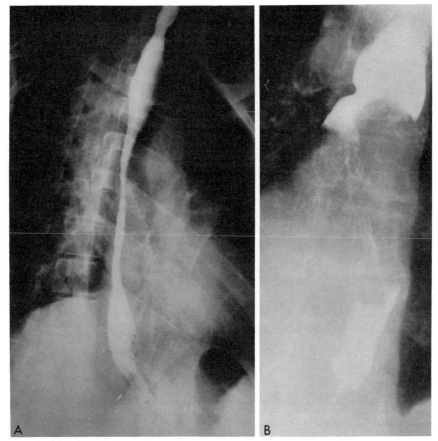

Figure 7–1. Compare the smoothly tapered appearance of a benign stricture *(A)* with the overhanging edges and destroyed mucosa of a cancer *(B)*. The lumen is almost totally obliterated by tumor growth.

definitely benign, (b) definitely malignant (if malignant, are there clues to histology? is it cancer or, for example, a lymphoma?), or (c) indeterminate (in this group are found lesions that cannot honestly be judged either benign or malignant. Further evaluation by another modality, such as endoscopy and biopsy, is necessary to make a definitive diagnosis).

NEOPLASMS OF THE GASTROINTESTINAL TRACT

The gastrointestinal tract can be thought of in general terms as a hollow, muscular tube. It is composed almost throughout its length of the same basic layers, which, if involved with neoplasm, will manifest a similar radiographic appearance regardless of the site. It is useful to think of neoplastic involvement of the GI tract

as being either intrinsic or extrinsic. Each will now be discussed separately.

Intrinsic Neoplasms

Intrinsic lesions arise from the layers of the gut itself. In simple terms, intrinsic involvement can be either *mucosal,* (arising from the mucosa and projecting into the lumen), *intramural* (arising from the submucosal layers and remaining largely confined to those layers), or *serosal* (Fig. 7–3).

A number of criteria enable the radiologist to distinguish between these. Lesions that are *pure*, i.e., solely mucosal, solely intramural, or solely extrinsic, can be differentiated by these criteria. If, however, the lesion involves more than one layer, e.g., an extrinsic lesion grows into the wall, it will appear as a combination of extrinsic and intramural lesions.

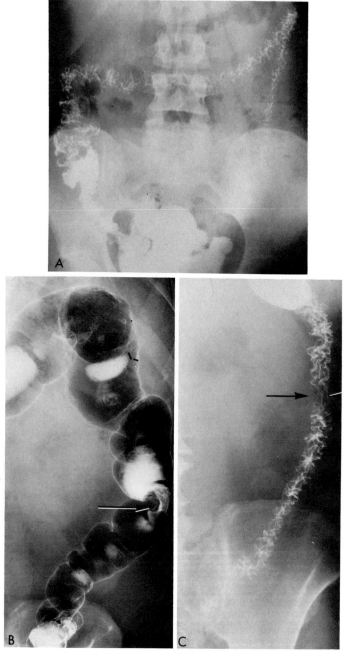

Figure 7–2. *A,* A normal postevacuation film shows the fine feathery mucosal pattern of the contracted colon. *B,* On this film of the well distended, barium-filled colon, there is a narrowed area in the descending colon (arrow); on this film it could be either benign or malignant. *C,* The postevacuation film shows that the mucosa in this area differs from the normal feathery pattern and does not contract normally. This region corresponds to the narrowed area on the distended film and this suspicious area must be evaluated further to exclude a tumor.

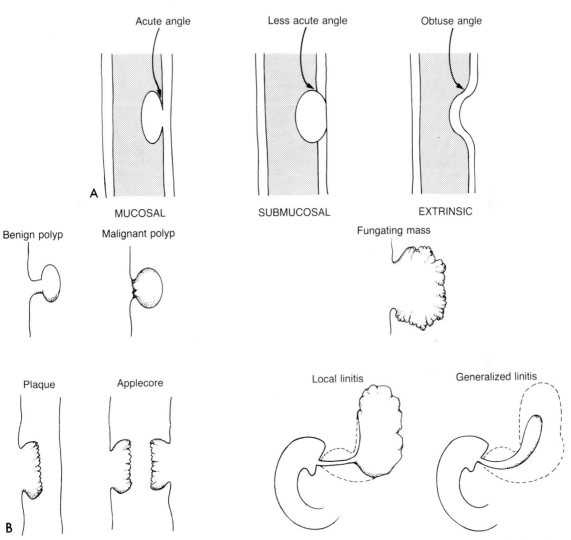

Figure 7–3. *A,* The abruptness of the junction of the lesion with normal bowel can help to localize the process as either intrinsic or extrinsic. A *mucosal* lesion makes an acute angle with surrounding bowel. The angle a *submucosal* lesion makes is less acute. A wholly *extrinsic* lesion smoothly indents the wall making a very obtuse angle. *B,* Line drawings of various forms of carcinoma of the bowel.

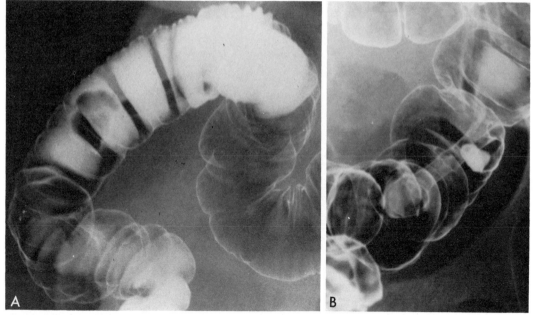

Figure 7–4. *A,* Polyp on a stalk; the lobulated polyp is seen as a negative filling defect within a positive pool of barium. *B,* On air contrast, the polyp is seen to be coated with barium and is therefore a filling defect etched in white. Incidentally note should be made of the pool of barium next to the stalk, which is a diverticulum filled with barium.

MUCOSAL LESIONS (POLYPS). The discussion of intrinsic neoplasms will begin by considering *mucosal* lesions, such as polyps. A polyp on a stalk is mobile to a certain extent; this mobility can be and should be radiographically demonstrable. A sessile polyp by definition "sits" on the mucosa, arises from a broad base, and is firmly attached to the mucosa; it is therefore immobile. To distinguish between these two categories, the radiologist must try to find the stalk if it is present. This is important, as sessile and pedunculated polyps have different implications and prognosis.

Either type of polyp will present as a negative shadow or filling defect in a column of contrast medium. With air contrast, thick barium coats the surface of the polyp, which will again be visible as a filling defect, but this time the defect will be of soft tissue density rimmed with white (adherent barium) in a column full of black (air) (Fig. 7–4).

Sometimes it is difficult to distinguish between a polyp and an empty diverticulum seen en face; of course if the diverticulum is seen in profile there is no problem. *Analysis of the ring will be helpful in this differentiation* (Fig. 7–5).

Polypoid lesions can occur anywhere along the length of the GI tract and will present a similar radiographic appearance no matter where they occur (Fig. 7–6). For the most part, this discussion will center on colonic polyps because they are so common. However, every radiologist will undoubtedly run across gastric or even small bowel polyps at

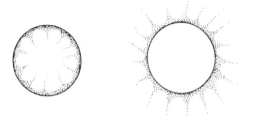

Figure 7–5. *Diverticulum viewed on end or polyp?* The diverticulum seen on end will have a sharp *outer* border and fade off centrally *(A).* The polyp seen en face will have a sharp *inner* border and fade off peripherally *(B).*

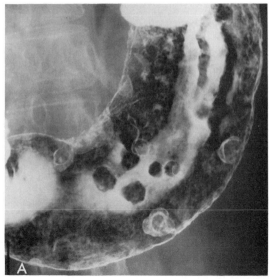

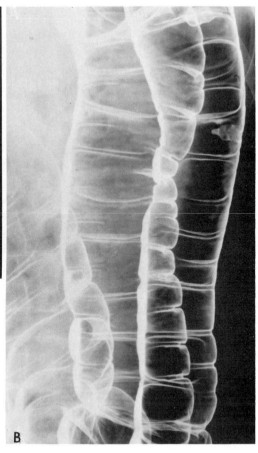

Figure 7–6. *Polyps. A,* Multiple gastric polyps are seen. Those on the posterior wall are round filling defects within a pool of barium; those on the anterior wall are sharp and "etched in white." Some of these are lobulated and may be adenomatous. That on the lesser curve has a puckered base and may be malignant. *B,* Notice the similarity of polyps of the colon to those of the stomach.

some time; the principles outlined for the colon can in general be applied in the others as well.

An important technical point to remember when performing single contrast studies is that polyps can be hidden by a large volume of contrast medium. Compression of the barium column (by a paddle, pressure cone, or the lead-gloved hand) displaces excess contrast around the lesion, rendering it visible again (Fig. 7–7). It is, however, possible to be overzealous: overcompression can make a lesion disappear because so much barium is pressed away that there is not enough left to coat it. Most radiologists consider the air contrast method superior for detecting small polypoid lesions, especially in anatomic areas where it is difficult to make use of compression (upper stomach, colonic flexures, rectum). In the best hands, a full-column enema will detect polyps in only 7 per cent of the population, compared

with 14 per cent with the air contrast technique; the latter figure approaches the incidence of polyps found at autopsy.

WHY LOOK FOR POLYPS? The majority of polyps (especially those less than 0.5 cm in size) are known to be hyperplastic and to have no malignant potential. In looking for polyps the search is for the adenoma, the polyp that may have malignant potential. How can the radiologist differentiate between these two types of polyps? In most cases, they cannot be distinguished. Hyperplastic and adenomatous polyps are essentially indistinguishable radiographically; they are simply filling defects in a contrast column. However, if the polyp is lobulated or large, it is more likely to be an adenoma.

In this regard, it is absolutely necessary to have a "clean colon." It has been shown that nearly 1 in 5 polypoidal colonic cancers were missed on a previous barium enema, not

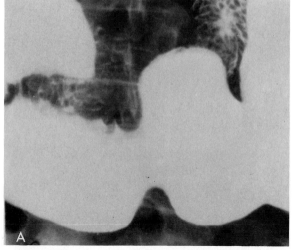

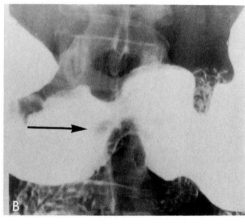

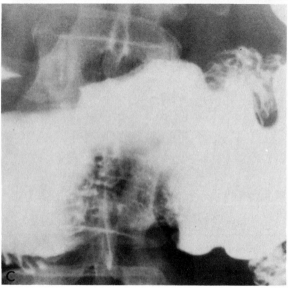

Figure 7–7. *Value of compression. A,* No polyp is seen without compression owing to the large amount of barium present. *B,* Graded compression makes the polyp visible (arrow) by pushing away the excess barium. *C,* If too much compression is applied, all the barium will be pushed away from around the polyp and it will no longer be seen.

because a filling defect was not seen, but because the defect was dismissed as stool! This is why you as a radiologist must insist on a clean colon and should not accept anything less.

Not all polyps are cancerous, therefore, but some cancers present as polyps. How can a polypoid lesion be judged on x-ray to be either benign or malignant?

Some criteria have been advanced to help distinguish benign from malignant lesions, and it is the radiologist's role to characterize each polyp.

1. *Sessile or pedunculated?* A polyp on a stalk is more likely to be benign than a sessile polyp. The stalk develops because the polyp begins as a mucosal lesion not fixed to the underlying submucosa; the fecal stream continually pulls at the polyp, stretching its base until a stalk forms. In theory, infiltrating tumor cannot be pulled along and remains locally adherent (i.e., sessile). It must be pointed out, however, that even some pedunculated polyps can be malignant or demonstrate carcinoma in situ (Fig. 7–8). This particularly applies to large polyps (but can be true

even of smaller ones): Again, the aim radiologically is to *find the stalk.*

2. *Size.* Once again it should be stressed that the majority of small polyps are benign, even if they are adenomas. The chance, however, that an adenomatous polyp is malignant increases the larger it is, from about 1 per cent for a 1 cm polyp to 25 per cent for a 2 cm polyp. Pedunculated polyps over 1.5 cm and sessile polyps over 1 cm should be considered potentially cancerous and biopsied. Small polyps were once dismissed as unthreatening, but recent experience has shown some of these are indeed malignant. Incidentally, because of magnification and other technical considerations, radiographic estimations of polyp size are not entirely accurate. For this reason, some believe all polyps should be biopsied or coagulated via colonoscopy.

3. *Base puckered or not?* Puckering of the base of a sessile polyp is an ominous sign, suggesting malignant invasion. Puckering of the base of a pedunculated polyp, however, can be brought about merely by the stalk pulling on the mucosa and is not a cause for concern.

4. *Surface.* A *smooth* surface suggests benignity; an irregular surface, malignancy.

One type of a polypoid lesion has certain

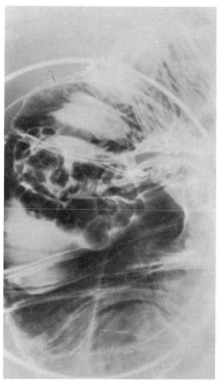

Figure 7–9. *Villous adenoma.* A large lobulated filling defect is seen within the ascending colon; barium has pooled in the interstices, which results in a frondlike pattern. This is the characteristic x-ray appearance of a villous adenoma.

pathologic features which result in a characteristic x-ray appearance: the villous tumor. Villous adenomas are made up of many fronds, and barium seeps into the interstices, resulting in an easily recognizable pattern (Fig. 7–9). Some 50 per cent of these are malignant, but even if benign, they can be debilitating because of profuse watery diarrhea. Note, however, that the mucus secretion from these tumors may be so high that they coat poorly and thus may easily be missed.

The importance of finding polyps is again emphasized. Whether or not cancers ultimately develop from adenomatous polyps has not been completely solved. However, many malignant neoplasms are polypoid, and it is impossible to tell malignant from benign polyps with certainty without a microscope. If, as many believe, cancers do arise from adenomatous polyps, it would certainly seem

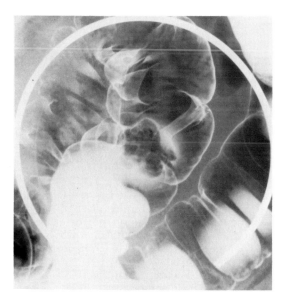

Figure 7–8. A 3 cm lobulated polyp is seen within the sigmoid colon. Although it is on a stalk, it was microscopically carcinoma in situ.

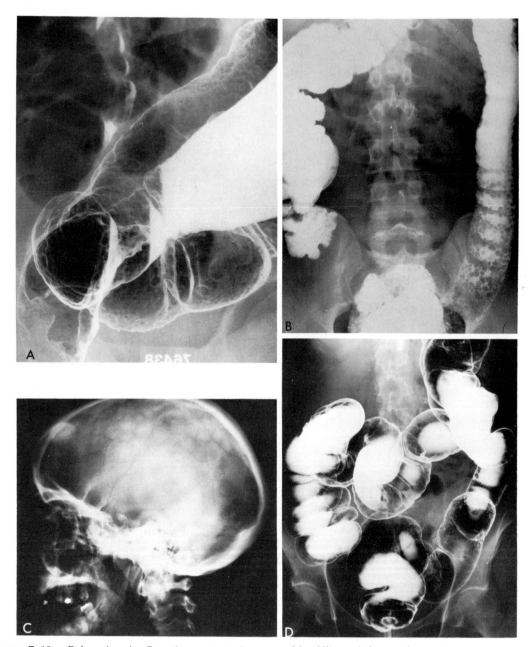

Figure 7–10. *Polyposis. A,* On air contrast innumerable filling defects of varying sizes are seen representing the polyps of familial polyposis. There is also irregularity of the right side of the rectum associated with a mass that was carcinoma. *B,* On full-column study innumerable polyps are visible (carpeting). (By courtesy of Deborah A. Hall, Massachusetts General Hospital, Boston.) *C,* A sclerotic area (an osteoma) is present in the frontal region on the skull x-ray of the same patient as in *B;* the combination of polyposis and osteomas is characteristic of Gardner's syndrome. *D,* Multiple filling defects are present throughout the colon, which might be confused with polyps. Note, however, that the defects are not round but irregular in shape and are due to adherent feces. This stresses the importance of a clean colon in diagnosing polyps.

wise to remove or at least to observe any polyps closely. This is particularly important not only because there is a relatively high incidence of adenomatous polyps but also because they are increasingly being found in younger people.

COLONOSCOPY OR BARIUM ENEMA? What is the best way to find or follow polyps? Colonoscopy is a good way of visualizing polyps, but it is cumbersome as a screening procedure. It is not 100 per cent accurate because of blind areas where the colon bends. In addition, it takes considerable expertise to reach the right colon. Although it used to be said that most carcinoma occurs in the rectum and sigmoid colon within reach of the sigmoidoscope, we seem to be finding an increasing number of cancers in the right colon, making the barium enema even more vital. Therefore, a reasonable polyp workup should include: air contrast barium enema followed by colonoscopy and biopsy of any polyps, especially those likely to be malignant. Follow-up air contrast barium enema and colonoscopy/biopsy should be performed as indicated; many recommend follow-up at 6 month or yearly intervals; a polyp that increases in size should be considered an aggressive lesion and biopsied.

POLYPOSIS. So far the discussion has concerned single polyps or at most a few individual polyps. Some people have many polyps; sometimes there are so many they are literally uncountable. These patients have one of the well-known polyposis syndromes, which include familial polyposis (Fig. 7–10), Gardner's syndrome, and Peutz-Jeghers syndrome. Although the features of these syndromes are conveniently summarized in Table 7–2, a brief description of each is in order here. Familial polyposis, Gardner's syndrome, and the rare Turcot's syndrome all involve primarily the colon; the polyps are adenomas. The most important reason to diagnose familial polyposis (and Gardner's syndrome) is the eventual development of colon cancer in these patients; patients with Turcot's syndrome ultimately develop central nervous system tumors. Family members of patients with familial polyposis or Gardner's syndrome should be screened after puberty when the polyps develop. Because of the bleak prognosis, many advocate prophylactic colectomy before 30 years of age. Patients with Peutz-Jeghers syndrome often come to attention because of their unusual mucocutaneous pigmentation. Peutz-Jeghers polyps are hamartomas rather than adenomas and tend to occur more in stomach and small bowel than in the colon. Intussusception may be the pre-

TABLE 7–2. POLYPOSIS SYNDROMES

	Heredity	Stomach	Small Bowel	Colon	Histology	Other Features	Associated Neoplasm
Familial polyposis	Dominant	<5%	<5%	100%	Adenoma		Colonic carcinoma
Gardner's	Dominant	5%	5%	100%	Adenoma	Soft tissue tumors Osteomas	Colonic carcinoma
Peutz-Jeghers syndrome	Dominant	25%	95%	30%	Hamartoma	Mucocutaneous pigmentation	Periampullary carcinoma ? Colonic carcinoma Ovarian tumors
Turcot's syndrome	Recessive	—	—	100%	Adenoma	CNS tumors	
Cronkhite-Canada syndrome	Not inherited	100%	50%	100%	Inflammatory	Alopecia, nail abnormalities, hyperpigmentation	

senting feature. Cronkhite-Canada syndrome is an unusual condition that occurs in a middle-aged to elderly population rather than the younger age group affected by the previously mentioned conditions; these polyps are inflammatory. Inflammatory polyps are also seen in juvenile polyposis; this disorder occurs in young children, and the polyps usually regress with time.

For all intents and purposes, Turcot's syndrome and Cronkhite-Canada syndrome are so rare that the radiologist is unlikely to see them in everyday practice.

Remember that other *high-risk groups* of patients exist (e.g., those with ulcerative colitis, patients with a family history of cancer or a previous history of polyps), to whom special attention must be paid.

INTRAMURAL (SUBMUCOSAL) NEO-PLASM. The second type of intrinsic neoplasm is the *intramural* or *submucosal* tumor. As with polypoid lesions, these can occur anywhere in the GI tract and be either benign or malignant. The radiographic appearance of a submucosal lesion is characteristic: a smooth, sharply outlined lesion covered by intact mucosa. The zone of transition between the lesion and surrounding normal tissue is broader (i.e., it make a less acute angle) than the abrupt origin of the mucosal lesion (acute angle); the edge of the lesion is therefore sharp and distinct.

Benign submucosal lesions include a wide variety of mesenchymal tumors, such as lipomas, leiomyomas, and neuromas, all of which have an identical radiographic appearance (Fig. 7–11), and biopsy is necessary to distinguish among them. Wherever they occur they appear the same on x-rays; an esophageal leiomyoma looks no different from a leiomyoma of the colon. Occasionally a colonic lipoma, frequently found at the ileocecal valve, may be differentiated from the others by a tap-water enema; the fat in the lipoma will then appear more translucent than the water in the colon.

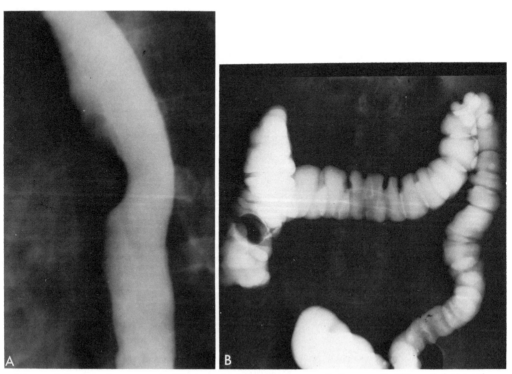

Figure 7–11. *Submucosal tumors. A,* Observe the sharply demarcated, smooth filling defect in the wall of the esophagus. Especially notice the relatively abrupt transition between the tumor and the esophagus itself indicating that this is an intramural lesion. *B,* A similar appearance is seen in the colon as a result of a lipoma of the valve.

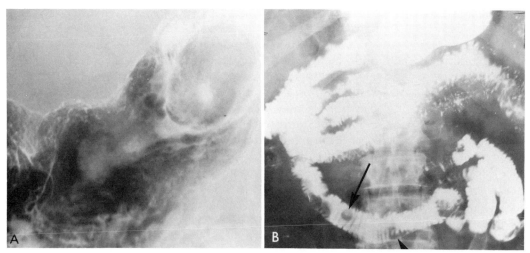

Figure 7–12. *A,* There is a well-circumscribed, sharply demarcated lesion with a central collection of barium in the fundus of the stomach; at surgery this was a leiomyoma with early carcinoma in situ. *B,* Multiple filling defects in small bowel with central collections of barium resulting in a target or "bull's-eye" appearance (arrows) are due to ulcerated metastases from malignant melanoma.

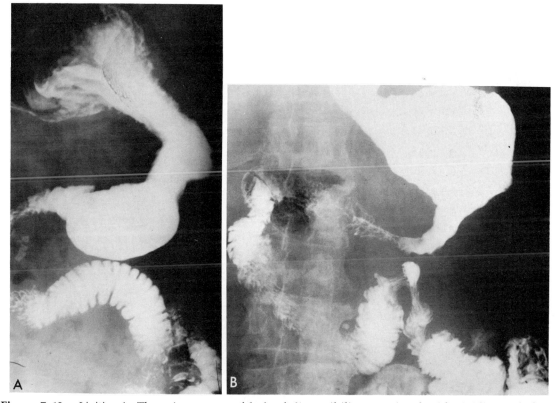

Figure 7–13. *Linitis. A,* There is an area of lack of distensibility associated with rigidity and sharp angulation in the midbody of the stomach; this was primary linitis plastica. *B,* Almost two thirds of the stomach is extremely narrowed and rigid, representing more diffuse linitis plastica.

The malignancy of these lesions may be difficult to assess; malignant submucosal tumors may be indistinguishable from their benign counterparts, and both benign and malignant tumors may ulcerate, resulting in a *target* or *bull's-eye* appearance (Fig. 7–12). Highly aggressive submucosal tumors may, however, have a "malignant" appearance, with infiltration and mucosal destruction. Very large ulcerated tumors in small bowel should suggest lymphosarcoma to the radiologist.

Not all submucosal processes are discrete nodules. Some highly malignant processes infiltrate the submucosal space diffusely and cause a narrowed, rigid appearance to the usually pliable viscus, resulting in the *"linitis plastica"* appearance (Fig. 7–13). This may occur anywhere in the gut but it is most common in the stomach. If the whole stomach is involved, the characteristic "leather bottle" appearance will result. Localized involvement may be more difficult to diagnose, but be alert to any narrowed, rigid, and nondistensible areas. This appearance may be due to a pri-

mary cancer, but certain metastases, e.g., from breast and lung, characteristically have this appearance as well. Because this tumor diffusely infiltrates the wall, early satiety is more likely to be the initial presentation than ulceration and bleeding.

SEROSAL NEOPLASM. Serosal involvement will result in spiculation, tethering, and sharp angulation of the loops involved (Fig. 7–14). Remember that although the classic appearance of serosal disease was described in the chapter on inflammatory diseases, neoplastic processes can affect the serosa in a similar fashion.

EXTRINSIC NEOPLASMS

Some neoplastic processes occur *external* to the gut; these include abdominal masses of all types, including many kinds of metastases. The radiographic appearance of a wholly *extrinsic* lesion is that of a *smooth, gently tapering defect* whose margins make an obtuse angle with the wall, as opposed to the more abrupt junction of an intramural lesion; it may also

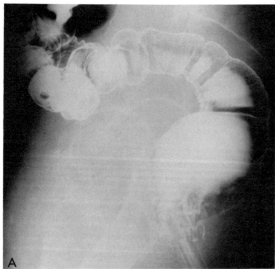

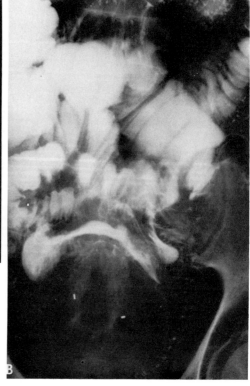

Figure 7–14. *Metastases. A,* There is spiculation and straightening of the anterior wall of the rectum due to a drop metastasis from a carcinoma of the hepatic flexure. Direct invasion of the serosa from a pelvic malignancy would have a similar appearance. *B,* Multiple loops with sharp angulation, fixation, and spiculation due to serosal metastases from carcinoma of the rectum.

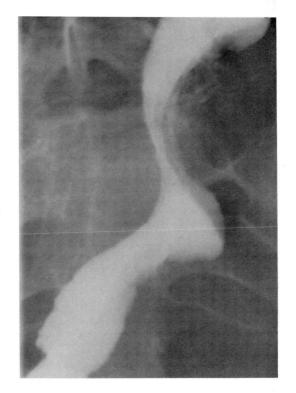

Figure 7–15. There is *extrinsic compression* on the rectosigmoid from large uterine fibroids. The characteristic appearance of an extrinsic lesion affecting the GI tract is shown; the indentation is smooth and broad and a double contour is present.

have a double contour. There should be no evidence of mucosal or submucosal involvement in a purely extrinsic lesion (Fig. 7–15). If the tumor invades the wall, however, the classic signs of extrinsic disease are lost, because the tumor has become partly intrinsic and will now show combined extrinsic and intrinsic characteristics.

Some common tumors will now be examined in more detail; remember that wherever they occur, tumors have a limited number of appearances, which depend on where the tumor originates and how it grows. The radiologist's aim is to recognize these abnormalities.

FINDINGS INDICATING NEOPLASTIC DISEASE

INFILTRATION. The involved area will not distend or change in shape with peristalsis

because it is rigid. This process may be localized to one wall forming a plaque, or it may encircle the bowel lumen resulting in the classic "napkin-ring" or "applecore" appearance. There will also be overhanging edges or shouldering due to tumor growth longitudinally.

MUCOSAL DESTRUCTION. The normal folds are either destroyed or replaced by an abnormal, distorted pattern.

MASS. A *mass* with or without ulceration is, of course, a characteristic appearance of tumor.

ESOPHAGUS

Carcinoma of the esophagus, a tumor which still has an extremely poor prognosis, is most commonly a *fungating* lesion (Fig. 7–16). Most are squamous cell lesions; a few are adenocarcinomas. Certain patients are particularly at

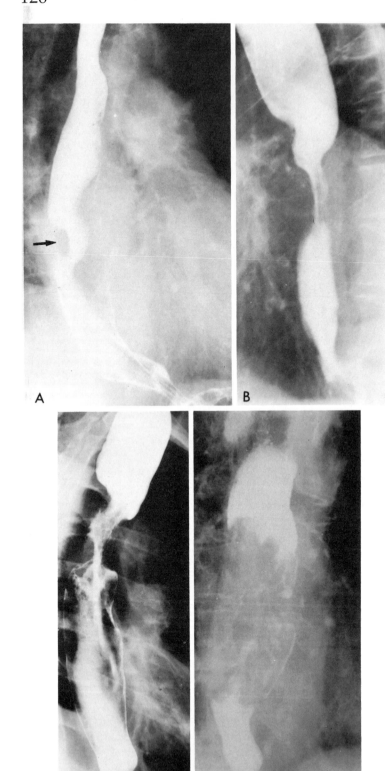

Figure 7–16. *The spectrum of carcinomas of the esophagus.*

A, On the posterior wall of the esophagus is a plaque-like lesion extending over a distance of approximately 2 cm, representing an early carcinoma (arrow).

B, The infiltrating variety; there is slight dilatation of the esophagus above the narrowed area, representing partial obstruction. Note that this infiltrating variety can be difficult to diagnose and even to separate from a benign lesion.

C, The annular constricting type with destruction of the mucosa and overhanging edges.

D, The polypoidal fungating variety with dilatation of the lumen around the tumor.

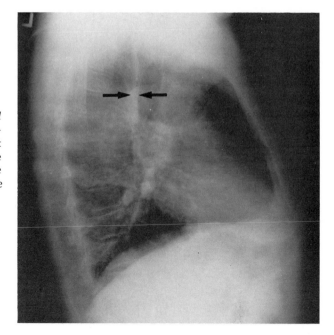

Figure 7–17. *Widening of the posterior tracheal stripe.* On this lateral chest x-ray, the posterior tracheal stripe is increased to almost 1 cm in width. (The normal posterior stripe has an upper limit of 3.5 mm.) This is the lateral chest x-ray from the patient whose barium swallow is seen in Figure 7–16C.

risk, especially those with a history of smoking or heavy alcohol consumption.

These carcinomas begin as sessile or plaque-like lesions limited to one wall and spread easily up and down the esophagus. Because the esophagus has no serosa, they easily invade the mediastinum, and the first hint of their presence can sometimes appear on a plain lateral chest film; the posterior tracheal stripe is widened beyond its normal upper limit of 3.5 mm (Fig. 7–17). Dysphagia characteristically is delayed until almost all of the lumen is encircled by tumor; a lesion which involves only part of the circumference will not result in dysphagia, as the remainder of the wall will distend to accommodate the bolus. The lesion is, therefore, usually well advanced when first documented by x-ray. The appearance on barium swallow can vary from a small plaque to an irregular shaggy stricture with overhanging edges to a large polypoid mass. Certain varieties tend to be especially bulky, such as the carcinosarcoma and the varicoid type. These tumors are easier to recognize than the diffusely infiltrating variety. Although the latter may appear frankly malignant, some may be no more than a region of indistensibility. For this reason any indistensible area should be carefully radiographed and suspicious ones biopsied.

Since the goal must be to detect potentially curable lesions, recently emphasis has been placed on detecting early superficial disease, which is best accomplished with the *air contrast technique.*

STOMACH

Carcinoma of the stomach is one of the few neoplasms to actually have shown a decreased incidence in the United States over the last 40 years. The disease process, however, is usually well advanced by the time diagnosis is made, and thus prognosis is poor. In Japan, where the incidence of gastric carcinoma is one of the highest in the world, much effort has been devoted to early diagnosis. In fact, Japanese radiologists popularized the double contrast study in the search for early gastric cancer; only in patients with this early lesion are survival data favorable.

The etiology of gastric carcinoma is unknown, but several conditions are associated with an increased incidence: adenomatous polyps, which may arise either de novo or following pernicious anemia or gastric resection. Disputed are associations with chronic peptic ulcer disease and chronic gastritis.

Cancer of the stomach occurs in several

different forms, and there are various systems of classification. The Japanese, who are probably most experienced with this disease, divide it into three basic groups. Type I consists of protruded lesions; type II of superficial lesions divided into subtypes (A, raised; B, flat; C, depressed); and type III of excavated lesions. These correspond well to pathologic classifications in common use in the United States: (1) polypoid (type I), (2) infiltrating (type II), and (3) ulcerating (type III).

Polypoid or fungating lesions vary in appearance from a solitary polyp to a bulky, cauliflower-like mass in which the mucosa is destroyed, resulting in absent or distorted folds. The adjacent gastric wall becomes stiffened and rigid, and peristalsis does not pass through this region.

Infiltrating tumor may be of two varieties: superficial spreading, localized to the mucosa or submucosa (seen in Japan), and the diffusely spreading or scirrhous type, also known as linitis plastica, which is more familiar to Western radiologists. In the more diffuse infiltrating type, the stomach wall is thickened, fibrotic, and rigid, and peristalsis does not pass through the abnormal area; this is demonstrated radiologically by noting that the shape of the stomach does not change (Fig. 7–18). The antrum is the most frequently involved site for the localized variety. The localized form can be extremely difficult to diagnose because the narrowing of the lumen caused by the thickened rigid wall may be subtle. This is why both coating and distention are so important in GI tract work. With the double contrast method, the radiologist can be particularly sure that there is actually lack of distention. The gas released should uniformly distend the stomach in the appropriate projection; any areas that do not distend are suspect.

No form of gastric cancer has raised more debate or caused as much confusion over its terminology than has the ulcerating variety. The debate has revolved around whether a simple benign gastric ulcer can become a cancer. Most believe gastric cancers are tumors from the very beginning and that they ultimately ulcerate as they outgrow their blood supply. It is obviously of great impor-

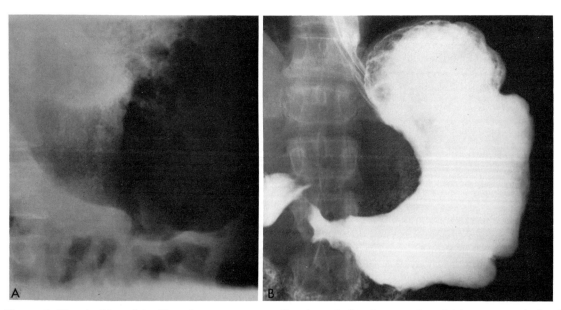

Figure 7–18. *A,* The plain film shows an unusually shaped distal stomach, which suggests lack of distensibility; note the fine calcifications. *B,* With contrast, the antrum and greater curvature of the stomach are thickened, rigid, and irregular, and the entire distal stomach is unchanging in shape. Incidentally, again note the calcification within the wall; this sandlike (psammomatous) calcification is characteristic of mucus-secreting adenocarcinoma, and both the primary tumor and the liver metastases may show the same features.

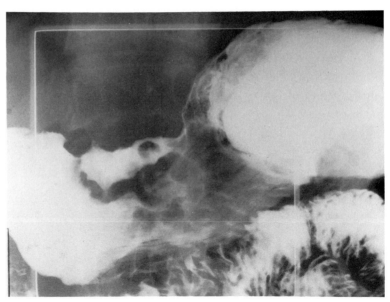

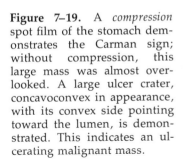

Figure 7–19. A *compression* spot film of the stomach demonstrates the Carman sign; without compression, this large mass was almost overlooked. A large ulcer crater, concavoconvex in appearance, with its convex side pointing toward the lumen, is demonstrated. This indicates an ulcerating malignant mass.

tance to distinguish "benign" from "malignant" ulcers. Most gastric ulcers (95 per cent) *are* benign; the radiologist's role is to properly diagnose the 5 per cent that are malignant. One semantic clarification: the ulcer *itself* is not malignant but occurs in a malignant tumor bed.

Several criteria have been proposed to differentiate benign from malignant ulcers. Remember that the ulcerating carcinoma is a mass in which an ulcer crater is located. Particular attention must be paid the area surrounding the ulcer for evidence of a tumor mass: heaped-up or nodular folds that stop short of the ulceration and a mass that projects into the lumen. Of historical interest is Carman's sign (Fig. 7–19). Carman and subsequent authors described the specific radiologic appearance of an ulcerating mass on the lesser curvature. This is a fluoroscopic finding seen only when the mass is compressed (see also Chapter 5).

DUODENUM AND SMALL BOWEL

Adenocarcinoma of the duodenum and small bowel is uncommon; the duodenum is more commonly involved by spread from adjacent organs, such as pancreas. Tumors involving the small bowel are more likely to be metastases or lymphomas than primary carcinoma,

and these will be discussed later in this chapter. When primary carcinoma does occur, it will have a similar appearance to carcinoma in other locations, i.e., an annular constriction with overhanging edges (Fig. 7–20).

COLON

Carcinoma of the colon, as already mentioned, accounts for a large percentage of cancer deaths in both men and women. Radiographic appearances are similar to those of the tumors already discussed.

These tumors are frequently polypoid and vary from a single polyp to a fungating mass. Large, broad-based polyps with surface irregularity suggest carcinoma. Since they are also intraluminal filling defects, they arise acutely from surrounding mucosa. Particularly in the cecum, they can grow quite large while remaining clinically silent; their only manifestation may be bleeding or anemia.

The infiltrating type of tumor is classic in appearance; it causes narrowing of the lumen, thickening of the wall, and rigidity. An annular "napkin-ring" or "applecore" appearance with mucosal destruction and overhanging edges results (Fig. 7–21). This type of colonic carcinoma is particularly prone to cause obstruction and may even perforate.

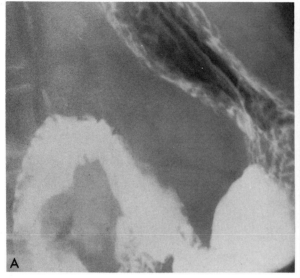

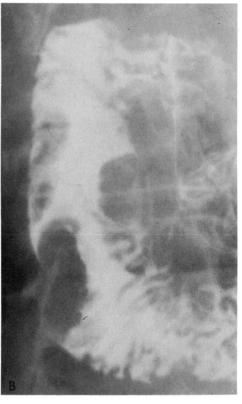

Figure 7–20. *A,* There is a *primary adenocarcinoma* of the second portion of the duodenum. (Courtesy of Dr. Stefan Schatzki, Mt. Auburn Hospital, Boston.) *B,* A close-up view of this tumor demonstrates the characteristic overhanging edges and applecore appearance of an annular constricting lesion.

TUMORS WITH PROTEAN MANIFESTATIONS

Metastases to the gut have many different appearances, depending on which layer they involve. They may reach the gut in three major ways and an understanding of these pathways will allow prediction of the radiographic appearance (Table 7–3). A consideration of this major problem will serve to summarize principles already discussed.

Pathways of Spread

Some tumors spread by direct extension from a primary tumor closely apposed to gut. This takes place most commonly in the confined pelvis, where tumors from either ovary, uterus, or prostate affect adjacent bowel, at first extrinsically and later submucosally as the tumor grows.

Another method is by direct extension from a primary tumor that is not immediately adjacent to the involved gut. Meyers (1975) has shown that the pathways of spread in-volve various mesenteries. Recollection of the anatomy will permit prediction of the site of spread. Thus, a gastric cancer can spread to the transverse colon. It will involve the *superior* surface because the gastrocolic ligament attaches superiorly to the transverse colon. On the other hand, pancreatic tumor will spread to the *inferior* surface of the transverse colon because the transverse mesocolon attaches *inferiorly* (Fig. 7–22). Initially serosal, the implants will change in appearance as they grow inward.

Meyers also discusses in detail the flow of ascitic fluid in the peritoneal cavity and shows how and where tumor cells, shed into this constantly circulating fluid, can implant. There are a number of favorite places for so-called "drop metastases." These are (1) pouch of Douglas, (2) the superior surface of the sigmoid colon, and (3) the right lower quadrant, including the terminal ileum and cecum. Incidentally, not only tumor cells but also any other substance released into the peritoneal fluid, such as pancreatic enzymes or therapeutic isotopes, will follow a similar path.

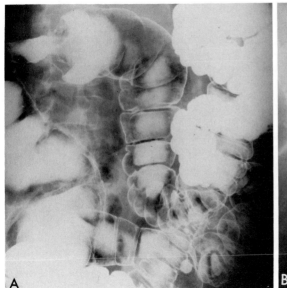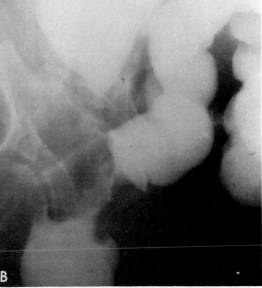

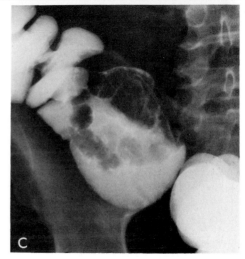

Figure 7–21. *Colon carcinoma. A,* An annular constricting lesion in the hepatic flexure, the classic "applecore" lesion of carcinoma, is seen. The central collection of barium indicates the lesion is ulcerating. *B,* A similar annular constricting carcinoma in the rectosigmoid colon. *C,* Not all carcinomas of the colon are of the annular constricting variety, and in this radiograph there is a large, irregular filling defect in the cecum with a central collection of barium; this is a large ulcerating polypoidal cancer.

TABLE 7–3. TUMORS THAT COMMONLY METASTASIZE TO THE GI TRACT

Primary Tumor	Spreads to	Route of Spread	Characteristic Radiographic Appearance
Melanoma	Stomach, small bowel, colon	Hematogenous	Nodules (target, bull's-eye)
Breast	Stomach, small bowel, colon	Hematogenous	Nodules or linitis
Lung	Stomach, small bowel, colon	Hematogenous	Nodules or linitis Mesenteric masses with angulation, etc.
Pancreas	Duodenum, colon	Direct extension	Serosal/submucosal
Colon	Stomach, small bowel	Seeding	Serosal/submucosal
Stomach	Small bowel, colon	Seeding	Serosal/submucosal
Ovary/Uterus	Small bowel	Seeding	Serosal/submucosal
Kidney	Colon	Direct extension to duodenum and descending colon, hematogenous	Serosal/submucosal, rarely bulky and intraluminal

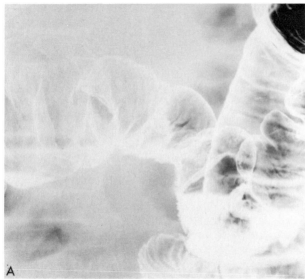

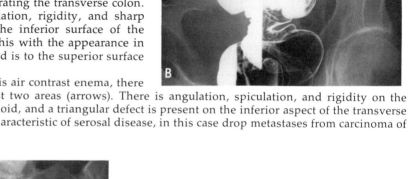

Figure 7–22. *A, Metastases to transverse colon from pancreatic carcinoma.* This is a coned-down view of an air contrast enema demonstrating the transverse colon. Serosal disease with spiculation, rigidity, and sharp angulation is evident on the inferior surface of the transverse colon. Contrast this with the appearance in Figure 1–5, where the spread is to the superior surface from gastric carcinoma.

B, Drop metastases. On this air contrast enema, there is serosal disease in at least two areas (arrows). There is angulation, spiculation, and rigidity on the superior surface of the sigmoid, and a triangular defect is present on the inferior aspect of the transverse colon. These findings are characteristic of serosal disease, in this case drop metastases from carcinoma of the pancreas.

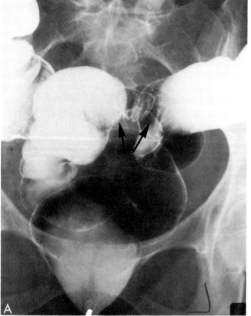

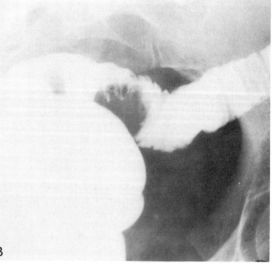

Figure 7–23. *Endometriosis.* Two ways in which endometriosis may manifest are shown. *A,* Initially it may appear as a smooth, eccentric, extrinsic defect (arrows) as shown here on the sigmoid colon. *B,* If the serosa is involved, there may be tethering and spiculation as well as the defect, indicating that this is not a totally extrinsic process.

132

The hematogenous route is the last important mode of spread. Again understanding this pathway will allow prediction of the x-ray appearance. Showers of tumor emboli reach the bowel via the arterial circulation and lodge in the submucosa. They will then have an appearance identical to that of a primary submucosal tumor, of either the infiltrating or the nodular variety. For instance, when breast cancer metastasizes to the stomach, as it frequently does, it characteristically presents as an infiltrating submucosal process indistinguishable from primary linitis plastica. Lung tumor and melanoma metastases, however, are frequently well-circumscribed submucosal nodules with central ulcerations, the well-known target lesions.

Endometriosis

An important differential consideration when evaluating a serosal or submucosal mass in a female is *endometriosis*, a quasi-neoplastic process. The endometrial implants may look exactly like metastatic serosal deposits (Fig. 7–23).

Carcinoid Tumors

Carcinoid tumors, the most common primary tumors of small bowel, can present either as intraluminal polypoid masses or as intramural nodules (Fig. 7–24); many are malignant. In the colon, the appendix is a favored location; here they are benign and usually occur as small nodules. In the right colon, they may present as large, fungating masses or applecore lesions, characteristically associated with a considerable desmoplastic response, which results in distortion and displacement of nearby bowel loops.

Lymphoma

Lymphoma likewise can have many different appearances, and as a consequence it is

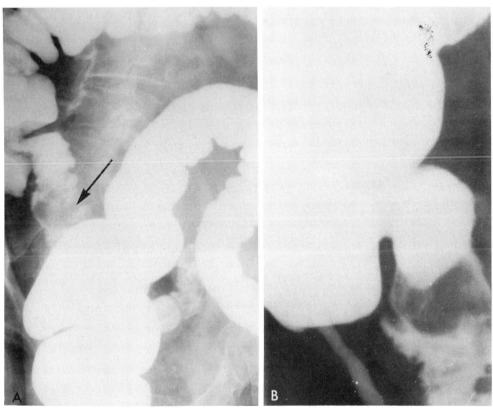

Figure 7–24. *Carcinoid. A,* A film of the terminal ileum shows a polypoidal filling defect (arrow), which is demonstrated better on the close-up view (*B*).

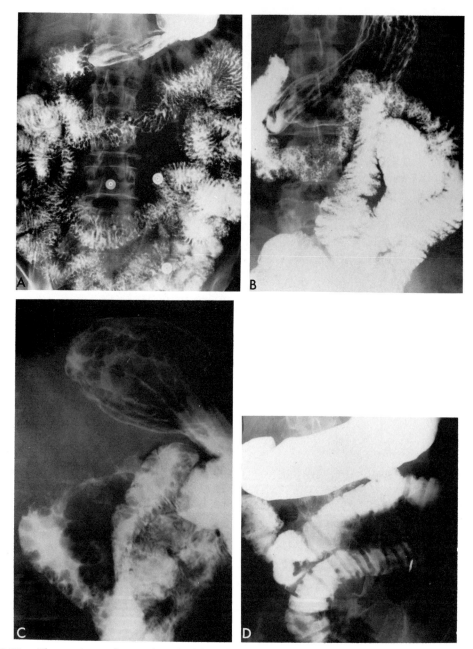

Figure 7–25. *The spectrum of gastrointestinal lymphoma.*

A, B, There are multiple *nodules* of varying sizes throughout the small bowel. Compare those in *A* with the nodules in *B,* which represent lymphoid hyperplasia; these are very tiny and of uniform size.

C, Multiple *nodules* of varying sizes are studded throughout the upper GI tract.

D and *E,* Fold thickening and nodules are seen throughout the small bowel. *E,* The fold thickening is even more obvious, and multiple submucosal nodular filling defects are present.

F, The *infiltrative* variety of lymphoma is demonstrated; there are two narrowed segments of small bowel with a characteristic appearance, known as "shaved mucosa" (arrows).

G, The large, irregular collection of barium with dilatation of the lumen and separation of bowel loops (arrow) is an ulcerating tumor. With this "aneurysmal dilatation" one should immediately think of lymphosarcoma.

H, This demonstrates the peculiar *endoexoenteric* form of lymphoma; this is categorized by multiple enteroenteric fistulous tracts and a large associated mass.

Illustration continued on opposite page

called the "great imitator." Marshak and others have described a variety of manifestations, running the gamut from nodules to ulcerating masses. Lymphoma may be either primary in the gut or secondary to involvement elsewhere. Some 15 per cent of patients who have lymphoma elsewhere in the body will have GI tract involvement, especially of stomach and small bowel, more rarely of the colon. The involvement may be (1) mucosal, with mass or ulceration; (2) submucosal, with thickened folds, mural infiltration, or nodules; (3) extrinsic defects due to masses in the mesentery; or (4) the unusual-appearing endoexoenteric mass that simulates Crohn's disease (Fig. 7–25). Aneurysmal dilatation of the lumen should immediately suggest lymphoma, as should "shaved mucosa." Lymphoma-

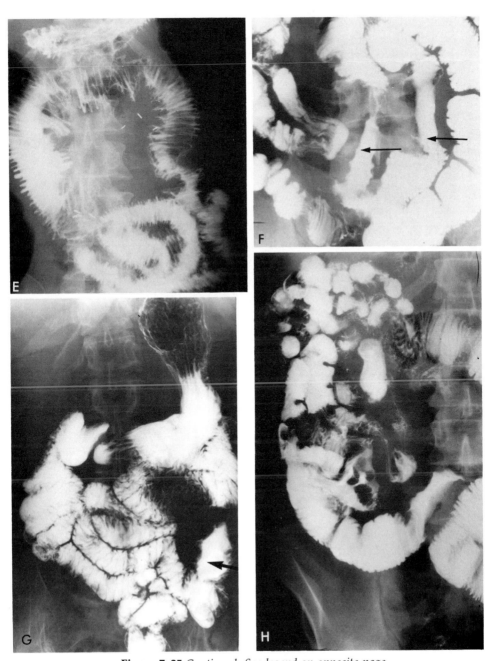

Figure 7–25 *Continued. See legend on opposite page*

tous involvement of the stomach is frequently submucosal and presents with thickened folds. In the small bowel, lymphoma may be more variable, presenting as thickened folds alone, nodules, or large ulcerating masses. Colonic lesions are less common but are essentially similar.

In concluding the discussion of lymphoma, it should be noted that some radiologists maintain they can distinguish between carcinoma and lymphoma, although in practice it is far more important to be able to tell malignant from benign processes than to try to distinguish between two malignancies. General criteria include the following: (1) lymphoma is softer, and thus more pliable than carcinoma, (2) it can transmit peristalsis, and so is not rigid, (3) it commonly spreads across the pylorus and ileocecal valve, which cancer rarely does, and (4) it should be suspected whenever thickened folds are seen anywhere in the GI tract. In practice, this distinction is not so easy to make, although sometimes lymphoma can be advanced as the more probable diagnosis. For example, a malignant gastric lesion associated with large folds suggests lymphoma rather than carcinoma, whereas a malignant ulcerating lesion in an atrophic stomach would suggest carcinoma as the more likely diagnosis.

References

Polyposis

Dodds WJ: Clinical and roentgen features of the intestinal polyposis syndromes. Gastrointest Radiol 1:127–142, 1976.
Dodds WJ, Lydon SB: Intestinal polyposis syndromes. CRC Crit Rev Clin Radiol 5:295, 1974.
Dodds WJ, Schulte WJ, Hensley GT, Hogan WJ: Peutz-Jeghers syndrome and gastrointestinal malignancy. Am J Roentgenol 115:374, 1972.
Godard JE, Dodds WJ, Phillips JC, Scanlon GT: Peutz-Jeghers syndrome: clinical and roentgenographic features. Am J Roentgenol 113:316, 1971.

Esophagus

Bachman AL, Teixidor HS: The posterior tracheal band: a reflector of local superior mediastinal abnormality. Br J Radiol 48:352–359, 1975.
Ital Y, Kogure T, Okuyama Y, Akiyama H: Superficial esophageal carcinoma: radiological findings in double-contrast studies. Radiology 126:597–601, 1978.
Koehler RE, Moss AA, Margulis AR: Early radiographic manifestations of carcinoma of the esophagus. Radiology 119:1, 1976.
Lindell MM Jr, Hill CA, Libshitz HL: Esophageal cancer: radio-

graphic chest findings and their prognostic significance. Am J Roentgenol 133:461, 1979.
Palayew MJ: The tracheo-esophageal stripe and the posterior tracheal band. Radiology 132:1:11, 1979.
Putman CE, Curtis AMcB, Westfried M, McLoud TC: Thickening of the posterior tracheal stripe: a sign of squamous cell carcinoma of the esophagus. Radiology 121:533–536, 1976.
Schatzki R, Haves LE: Roentgenologic appearance of extramucosal tumors of esophagus. Am J Roentgenol 48:1, 1942.
Yates CW Jr, LeVine MA, Jensen KM: Varicoid carcinoma of the esophagus. Radiology 122:605–608, 1977.

Stomach

Ferrucci JT Jr, Janower ML: Localized infiltrating lesions of the stomach. Semin Roentgenol 6:168, 1971.
Kirklin BR: The meniscus-complex in the roentgenologic diagnosis of ulcerating carcinoma of the stomach. Am J Roentgenol 47:571–577, 1942.
Koga M, Nakata H, Kiyonari H, Inakura M, Tanaka M: Roentgen features of the superficial depressed type of early gastric carcinoma. Radiology 115:289, 1975.
Marshak RH, Lindner AE: Polypoid lesions of the stomach. Semin Roentgenol 6:151, 1971.
Ming SC: Malignant potential of gastric polyps. Gastrointest Radiol 1:121–125, 1976.
Shirakabe, H: Atlas of X-ray Diagnosis of Early Gastric Cancer. Philadelphia, JB Lippincott, 1966.

Colon

Dreyfuss JR, Benacerraf B: Saddle cancers of the colon and their progression to annular carcinomas. Radiology 129:289–293, 1978.
Felson B (Ed): Localized solitary lesions of the colon. Semin Roentgenol II:2, 1976.
Gabrielsson N, Granqvist S, Ohlsen H, Sundelin P: Malignancy of colonic polyps: diagnosis and management. Acta Radiol Diagn 19:479, 1978.
Htoo AM, Bartram CI: The radiological diagnosis of polyps in the presence of diverticular disease. Br J Radiol 52:263–267, 1979.
Lane N, Fenoglio CM: Observations on the adenoma as precursor to ordinary large bowel carcinoma. Gastrointest Radiol 1:111–119, 1976.
Leinicke JL, Dodds WJ, Hogan WJ, Stewart ET: A comparison of colonoscopy and roentgenography for detecting polypoid lesions of the colon. Gastrointest Radiol 2:125–128, 1977.
Miller RE, Lehman G: Polypoid colonic lesions undetected by endoscopy. Radiology 129:295–297, 1978.
Ott DJ, Gelfand DW: Colorectal tumors: pathology and detection. Am J Roentgenol 131:691–695, 1978.

Neoplasms with Protean Manifestations

Balthazar EJ: Carcinoid tumors of the alimentary tract. I. Radiographic diagnosis. Gastrointest Radiol 3:47–56, 1978.
Bancks NH, Goldstein HY, Dodd GD: The roentgenologic spectrum of small intestinal carcinoid tumors. Am J Roentgenol 123:274–280, 1975.
Banner MP, Gohel VK: Peritoneal mesothelioma. Radiology 129:637–640, 1978.
Berk RN, Scher GS, Bode DF: Unusual tumors of the gastrointestinal tract. Am J Roentgenol 113:159, 1971.
Fagan CJ: Endometriosis: clinical and roentgenographic manifestations. Radiol Clin North Am 12:109, 1974.
Kinkhabwala M, Balthazar EJ: Carcinoid tumors of the alimentary tract. II. Angiographic diagnosis of small intestinal and colonic lesions. Gastrointest Radiol 3:57–62, 1978.
Lazarus H, Widrich WC, Robbins AH: Peritoneal mesothelioma with roentgenographic findings. Am J Roentgenol 113:171, 1971.
Stein LA, Margulis AR: The spheroid sign: a new sign for accurate

differentiation of intramural from extramural masses. Am J Roentgenol 123:420, 1975.

Zollinger RM: Cannon lecture: islet cell tumors and the alimentary tract. Am J Roentgenol 126:5:933, 1976.

Metastases

Chang SF, Burrell MI, Brand MH, Garsten JJ: The protean gastrointestinal manifestations of metastatic breast carcinoma. Radiology 126:611–617, 1978.

Ginaldi S, Lindell MM Jr, Zornoza J: The striped colon. A new radiographic observation in metastatic serosal implants. Am J Roentgenol 134:453–456, 1980.

Goldstein HM, Beydoun MT, Dodd GD: Radiologic spectrum of melanoma metastatic to the gastrointestinal tract. Am J Roentgenol 129:605, 1977.

Meyers MA: Metastatic seeding along the small bowel mesentery: Roentgen features. Am J Roentgenol 123:67–73, 1975.

Meyers MA, McSweeney J: Secondary neoplasms of the bowel. Radiology 105:1–11, 1972.

Oddson TA, Rice RP, Seigler HF, Thompson WM, Kelvin FM, Clark WM: The spectrum of small bowel melanoma. Gastrointest Radiol 3:419, 1978.

Smith SJ, Carlson HC, Gisvold JJ: Secondary neoplasms of the small bowel. Radiology 125:29–33, 1977.

Lymphoma

Balikian JP, Nassar NT, Shamma'a MH, Shahid MJ: Primary lymphomas of the small intestine including the duodenum: a roentgen analysis of twenty-nine cases. Am J Roentgenol 107:131–141, 1969.

Brady LW, Asbell SO: Malignant lymphoma of the gastrointestinal tract. Erskine Memorial Lecture, 1979. Radiology 137:291, 1980.

Carnovale RL, Goldstein HM, Zornoza J, Dodds GD: Radiologic manifestations of esophageal lymphoma. Am J Roentgenol 128:751–754, 1977.

Chiles JT, Platz CE: The radiographic manifestations of pseudo-lymphoma of the stomach. Radiology 116:551, 1975.

Dunnick NR, Harell GS, Parker BR: Multiple "bull's-eye" lesions in gastric lymphoma. Am J Roentgenol 126:965–969, 1976.

Hricak H, Thoeni RF, Margulis AR, Eyler WR, Francis IR: Extension of gastric lymphoma into the esophagus and duodenum. Radiology 135:309–312, 1980.

Marshak RH, Lindner AE, Maklansky D: Lymphoreticular disorders of the gastrointestinal tract: roentgenographic features. Gastrointest Radiol 4:103–120, 1979.

Menuck LS: Gastric lymphoma, a radiologic diagnosis. Gastrointest Radiol 1:157–161, 1976.

O'Connell DJ, Thompson AJ: Lymphoma of the colon: the spectrum of radiologic changes. Gastrointest Radiol 2:377–385, 1978.

Zornoza J, Dodd GD: Lymphoma of the gastrointestinal tract. Part II. Semin Roentgenol 15:272, 1980.

8

SMALL BOWEL

THE SMALL BOWEL FOLLOW-THROUGH

A multitude of diseases can affect the small bowel, so the radiologist will often be asked to perform a small bowel series (small bowel follow-through). Unfortunately, this study has a bad reputation; many perform it in a perfunctory fashion, as an afterthought to an upper GI series. To do this study properly, however, careful monitoring is needed, or large segments of bowel may not be seen. A common mistake is to wait too long before taking the first film, allowing most of the barium to reach the distal small bowel. Each study must be tailored to the individual patient; how many films and the interval between films depend on the transit time and whether any abnormality is seen. Any suspicious areas on the overhead films should be fluoroscoped immediately and compression spot films obtained. Because a large number of diseases involve the terminal ileum, spot films with compression of this area should be performed if possible in every patient (unless this area is seen exceptionally well on the overhead films).

Even with careful monitoring, however, the rate of identifying pathologic lesions in the small bowel is low compared with that for the remainder of the gastrointestinal tract. There are a number of reasons for this. The small bowel, because it is extremely long and makes multiple convoluted turns, is extremely difficult to study. Even with compression (films are taken with the patient prone), overlapping loops are a problem, especially low in the pelvis. It is important to maintain a continuous column of barium; otherwise adequate distention will not be obtained, and

lesions will be missed (Fig. 8–1). Even with 2 cups (16 oz) of barium and the patient lying on the right side to facilitate gastric emptying, adequate distention may be difficult to obtain; if the column breaks up or the bowel is contracted, lesions will be missed.

Although the average time for barium to reach the cecum is not exorbitant (45 minutes to 1½ hours), in some patients a small bowel follow-through seems to take forever; how quick the study is (and therefore how many and how often films need to be taken) depends on the speed of transit. Many drugs and diseases (diabetes, sprue, scleroderma) will slow down small bowel motility, and the study will then take several hours, taxing both the patient's and the radiologist's patience. To avoid a disgruntled patient, you should tell the patient that you will be following the barium through to the colon and that how long the study takes depends on his or her intestines. Some tricks may help speed the study: a glass of iced water or food will help once the barium reaches the ileum. Ten to 20 ml of Gastrografin added to the barium will stimulate peristalsis but may result in dilution, so this is not a good idea if the question is malabsorption. Various drugs have been used (neostigmine, metoclopramide), but none has gained widespread use. Interestingly, glucagon, after initially paralyzing the bowel, seems to have a rebound effect, speeding transit considerably.

What barium preparation should be used? Many are available, some making claims to be better for the small bowel than others, some claiming to speed transit by having sorbitol and water-soluble contrast medium already in them. Basically, however, a good UGI barium should be an all-purpose

138

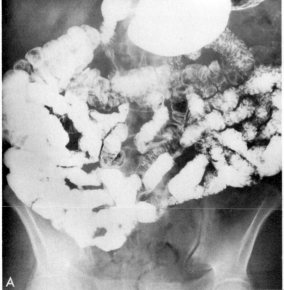

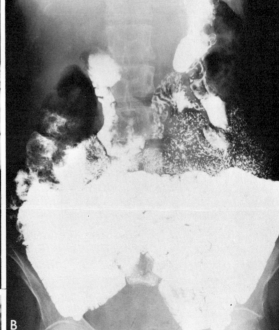

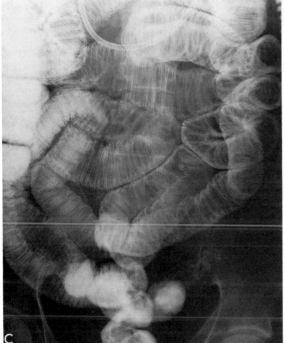

Figure 8–1. *Small bowel series. A,* With a small bowel follow-through, there are some underdistended and other underpenetrated loops. *B,* The loops are also somewhat overlapping, particularly evident here, with at least three quarters of the small bowel being overlapped, underpenetrated, underdistended, and basically unsatisfactorily examined. Even with compression, many loops would not be seen and lesions will be missed.

C, Enteroclysis. By distending the loops, the problem of overlapping is overcome. Although compression does play a part in this technique, it is primarily a "see-through" examination.

one and should allow study of both the stomach and the small bowel at the same sitting if desired.

Enteroclysis

Enteroclysis (the small bowel enema) has overcome some of the problems inherent in the regular small bowel follow-through. It is, however, a time-consuming (and somewhat unpleasant) procedure, which involves passing a nasogastric tube and then positioning it through the pylorus and around to the ligament of Treitz. Barium, or barium followed by water or methyl cellulose to give a double contrast effect, is infused at a rate fast enough

TABLE 8–1. A SIMPLE APPROACH TO SMALL BOWEL DISEASE

1. Transit Time

Prolonged	*Shortened*
Ileus	Anxiety and tension
Obstruction	Thyrotoxicosis
Scleroderma	Drugs: Metoclopramide (Reglan)
Drugs: Morphine	Quinidine
Lomotil	Mecholyl
Atropine	Neostigmine
Pro-Banthine	
Vagotomy	

2. Size

Dilated	*Contracted*
Ileus	Underfilling
Obstruction	Carcinomatosis
Sprue	
Scleroderma or other diseases that destroy smooth muscle, e.g., lymphoma	
Drugs	Drugs (as above)
(same as those that prolong transit)	

3. Fold Pattern

Normal	*Thick (Stack-of-Coins)*	*Thick and Distorted*
Ileus	Submucosal hemorrhage (ischemia)	Infiltrating disease
Obstruction	Submucosal edema (hypoproteinemia, radiation, inflammation)	Lymphoma
Sprue		Whipple's disease (especially in jejunum)
		Immunoglobulin deficiency
		Lymphangiectasia
		Giardiasis
		Amyloid

4. Nodules

Small to Medium Size	*Variable Size*
Lymphoid hyperplasia	Lymphoma
Infiltrating diseases	Metastases
Diseases of the lymphoid tissue	
Immunoglobulin deficiency states	
Macroglobulinemia	

to distend the bowel. Thus, the problems of overlapping loops and inadequate distention are less, but compression and oblique views are still necessary to separate all the loops.

Many believe that study of the small bowel should begin with a regular small bowel series and proceed to enteroclysis only if the conventional study is *negative*. In malabsorption a small bowel follow-through may be diagnostic. However, in a patient with unexplained GI blood loss and normal UGI series small bowel follow-through and barium enema, enteroclysis may find the lesion. Proponents of enteroclysis claim that the regular small bowel follow-through is so inaccurate that all studies of the small bowel should be performed by this method. Certainly it can

pick up and define much pathology that has not been demonstrated in a small bowel follow-through.

Interpreting the Study

The seemingly endless list of diseases that may affect the small bowel usually overwhelms the casual observer. There are, however, a number of basic principles, which allow a simple analysis of small bowel disorders and make this topic less frightening (see Table 8–1).

When observing a small bowel series, try to follow a sequence, such as the following:

1. Is the bowel dilated or not? Are there any narrowed areas?

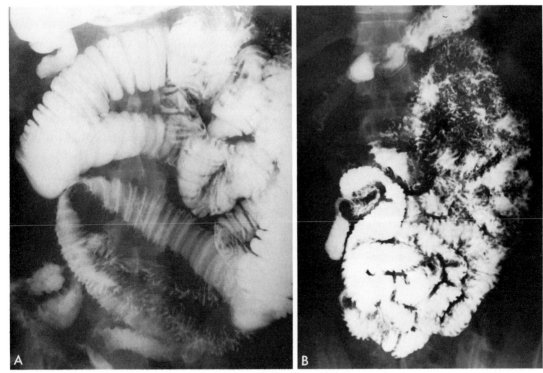

Figure 8–2. *Fold thickening. A,* Compare the fold pattern in the proximal small bowel with that occurring more distally. Proximally there is dilatation with a normal fold pattern due to a partial obstruction distally. In the mid–small bowel there is marked fold thickening in a "stack-of-coins" or "picketfence" appearance associated with luminal narrowing and wall thickening. This regular fold thickening is characteristic of submucosal fluid and is therefore the appearance in ischemia, bleeding, or inflammation. In this patient it was due to ischemia.

B, Amyloidosis. There is marked abnormality affecting the jejunum and relative sparing of the ileum. The abnormality consists of marked thickening of the small bowel folds in an irregular fashion in comparison with the regular thickening in *A.* This indicates some form of infiltrating disease.

2. What do the folds look like?
3. Are there any nodules?
4. Is the wall thick?
5. Is there any evidence of mass lesions?
6. Are there any changes in the barium?

Changes in Barium

The changes in the barium are usually obvious, so they will be discussed first. Modern barium preparations are chemically stable, remaining liquid and in a continuous column in the normal small bowel. In the presence of excess intraluminal fluid (e.g., malabsorption), however, the barium will undergo some chemical change; in such cases *dilution, flocculation* (barium breaking up into small flecks), and *segmentation* (the column of barium fragmenting, resulting in large globs) will be seen.

Is the Bowel Dilated?

The normal diameter of the lumen is 25 to 30 mm, roughly the size of a quarter. Dilatation may be associated with a number of processes, e.g., obstruction or ileus, motility or muscle disorders, sprue, and ingestion of many drugs.

Is the Fold Pattern Normal?

Normal folds (with contrast, these are the *translucencies* crossing the bowel) are fine and feathery, relatively straight, and 2 to 3 mm thick. Many diseases can result in fold thickening, which may be either regular or irregular (Fig. 8–2).

REGULAR THICKENING. With *regular* thickening, each fold is abnormal but still straight, resulting in a "stack-of-coins" or "picketfence" appearance. This is due to submucosal fluid of any kind, such as blood or edema. Ischemia, hemorrhage, or inflammation — for example, from radiation damage — will all give this pattern; the difference cannot be decided radiologically without some clinical correlation.

IRREGULAR THICKENING. When *irregularly thickened*, the fold pattern is distorted, the folds running in many different direc-

tions. This usually indicates an infiltrating disease (such as amyloid or Whipple's disease) or disease of lymphoid tissue (lymphoma, lymphangiectasia, immunoglobulin deficiency, giardiasis).

Sometimes the appearance is hard to categorize, but then the radiologist should try to choose a characteristic area and not be led astray by one small area that does not fit into the general picture.

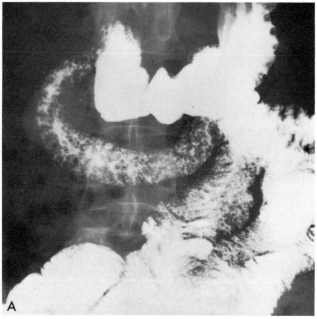

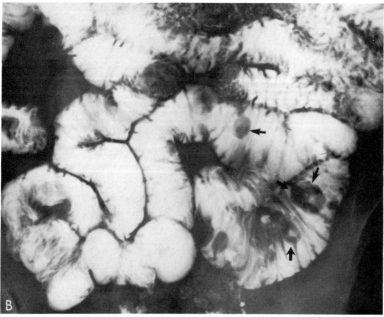

Figure 8–3. *A, Lymphoid hyperplasia.* Multiple tiny nodular filling defects are seen within the duodenal C-sweep and proximal jejunum. These sandlike nodules represent hyperplastic lymph follicles (lymphoid hyperplasia).

B, Metastatic melanoma. There are multiple round filling defects of varying sizes (arrows), many of which have central ulceration. This appearance is highly characteristic of metastatic melanoma and Kaposi's sarcoma.

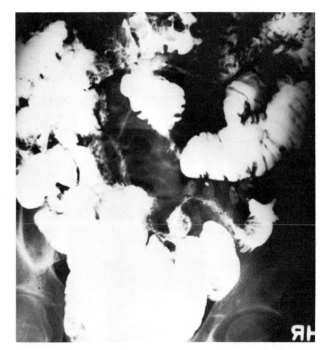

Figure 8–4. *Crohn's disease with marked bowel wall thickening.* There are multiple "skip" areas in which there is luminal narrowing, spiculation, and nodularity; the bowel loops are widely separated, indicating bowel wall thickening.

Are There Any Nodules Present?

If so, are these tiny or large? Do they vary in size? Are any of them ulcerated? Sometimes whether there are nodules or not is easy to decide, sometimes it is difficult. It is important not to confuse folds viewed on end with real nodules. If there is doubt, nodules are probably not present. In general, nodules are associated with any infiltrating disease or one which affects the lymphoid tissue of the small bowel (Fig. 8–3). Hematogenous metastases may also be nodules. Characteristically, since these result from different seedings, metastatic nodules vary in size; they lodge in the submucosa, where the nutrient arteries perforate the bowel wall. At post mortem, small bowel metastases are common, especially from such tumors as melanoma or breast or lung cancers. Occasionally these metastases have a central ulceration or dimple, resulting in the classic "bull's-eye" or "target" appearance; this is the characteristic appearance of metastases from malignant melanoma or Kaposi's sarcoma. Metastases from lung or breast cancers may also present as small bowel nodules, although a favorite place for breast metastases is the stomach, where it simulates linitis plastica.

WALL THICKNESS AND EVIDENCE OF MASS LESIONS WITHIN THE MESENTERY. Normal small bowel loops should be close together, separated by only a few millimeters, the thickness of two adjacent walls. Any infiltrative process, such as inflammation, bleeding, or tumor, will thicken the bowel wall and the abnormal loops will appear further apart than usual (Fig. 8–4).

Ascites will also cause loops to appear separated, because any gas-filled loops will float in the fluid. Even more marked displacement of small bowel loops will occur if there is a mass in the mesentery.

At the same time, each bowel loop should be smoothly undulating. Remember, sharp curves and straight lines do not belong on radiographs of the abdomen. Any abrupt angulation indicates that a loop is *tethered* and unable to move; this may result from either an inflammatory or a malignant process.

Incidentally, small bowel abnormalities can be further characterized by which border, mesenteric or antimesenteric, the process affects. Most diseases (Crohn's disease, lymphoma, seeded metastases) involve the mesenteric side of the loop; hematogenous metastases and Meckel's diverticulum involve the opposite, antimesenteric side.

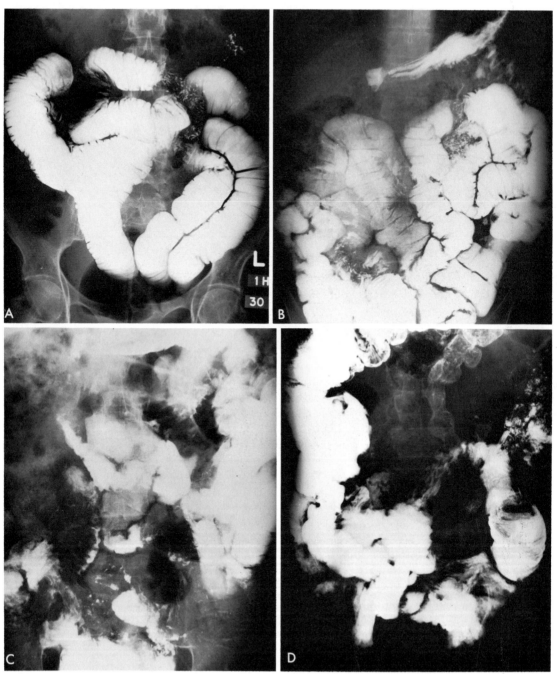

Figure 8–5. *The many faces of sprue. A,* There is dilatation with a normal or slightly less obvious fold pattern. *B,* In addition to dilatation of small bowel, as in *A,* this patient demonstrates dilution of the barium due to excess of intraluminal fluid. *C,* As the study proceeds, segmentation and flocculation become more evident. The fold pattern is now very difficult if not impossible to characterize. *D,* Even later a markedly dilated loop is seen in the left lower abdomen, which contains a filling defect. This has the characteristic coiled-spring appearance of an intussusception.

It might seem from the foregoing that specific diagnoses are easy. Occasionally the specific diagnosis *is* obvious — e.g., target metastases. It should be understood, however, that with small bowel disease a specific diagnosis often cannot be made. Instead, a differential diagnosis must be offered. The clinical picture, laboratory studies, and small bowel biopsy will help to clarify those cases in which the findings are not specific.

In some diseases, the small bowel series is normal unless the patient is stressed. This is seen especially in deficiency states, such as lactase or disaccharidase deficiency, in which the small bowel follow-through becomes abnormal only if the offending agent is added to the barium. The addition of lactose (50 grams) to barium in a patient with lactase deficiency will result in extremely rapid transit, abdominal cramping, diarrhea, and dilution of the barium. This is a positive stress test.

MALABSORPTION

Malabsorption is a feature of many diseases. Sometimes it is possible only to say (from seeing dilution, flocculation, and perhaps segmentation) that the patient has malabsorption; at other times a *specific diagnosis* can be made (e.g., jejunal diverticulosis).

SPRUE

Sprue (adult celiac disease, gluten-sensitive enteropathy, nontropical sprue) is one of the diseases of malabsorption which in general is underdiagnosed. The radiologist, however, can be one of the first to suggest this diagnosis, which can then be confirmed by small bowel biopsy. In tropical sprue, the findings may be identical but there will be a history of living in the tropics; the characteristic response of tropical sprue to tetracycline helps to separate tropical from nontropical sprue.

Findings on small bowel follow-through that should suggest the diagnosis of sprue are the following (Fig. 8–5):

1. *Dilatation*. A constant feature, presumably due to a combination of muscle weakness and the increase in intraluminal fluid.

2. *Dilution*, flocculation, and segmentation. A specific appearance is "moulage;" the barium looks like wax poured into a featureless mold of the intestine.

3. The *folds* are usually normal or thinner than usual, although they may appear thickened in cases of marked hypersecretion.

4. *Intussusception*. A transient, self-reducing intussusception (the classic "coiled-spring" appearance) may be seen during the small bowel series. In a patient with malabsorption, this should suggest sprue. Why this occurs is not known, but it is thought to account in part for the cramping abdominal pain these patients experience.

5. *Duodenal ulcerations*. Ulcers of the C-sweep or small bowel in association with malabsorption are characteristic (if rare).

6. *Transit time* may be normal or, more characteristically, prolonged.

Occasionally patients with sprue will relapse despite a gluten-free regimen; in these people, one should immediately suspect *lymphoma*, the incidence of which is increased in sprue. It has also been realized recently that there is an increased risk of GI malignancy in general in this disease, and sprue is now considered a *premalignant condition*.

References

General

Goldberg HI, Sheft DJ: Abnormalities in small intestine contour and caliber, a working classification. Radiol Clin North Am 14:461–476, 1976.

Marshak RH, Lindner AE: Radiology of the Small Intestine. 2nd Ed. Philadelphia, WB Saunders Co, 1976.

Osborn AG, Friedland GW: A radiological approach to the diagnosis of small bowel disease. Clin Radiol 24:281–301, 1973.

Sellnik JL: Radiological Atlas of Common Diseases of the Small Bowel. Leiden, Netherlands, Stenfert Kroese BV, 1976.

Tully TE, Feinberg SB: A roentgenographic classification of diffuse diseases of the small bowel intestine presenting with malabsorption. Am J Roentgenol 121:283–290, 1974.

Enteroclysis

Miller RE, Sellink JL: Enteroclysis: the small bowel enema. Gastrointest Radiol 4:269–283, 1979.

Anatomy

Balthazar EJ, Gade MF: Gastrointestinal edema in cirrhotics. Gastrointest Radiol 1:215–223, 1976.

Dalinka MK, Wunder JF: Meckel's diverticulum and its complications with emphasis on roentgenologic demonstration. Radiology 106:295, 1973.

Meyers MA: Clinical involvement of mesenteric and antimesenteric borders of small bowel loops. I. Normal pattern and relationships. II. Radiologic interpretation of pathologic alterations. Gastrointest Radiol 1:41–58, 1976.

Malabsorption

Collins SM, Hamilton JD, Lewis TD, Laufer I: Small bowel malabsorption and gastrointestinal malignancy. Radiology 126:603–609, 1978.

Isbell RG, Carlson HC, Hoffman HN II: Roentgenologic-pathologic correlation in malabsorption syndromes. Am J Roentgenol 107:158–169, 1969.

Marshak RH, Lindner AE: Malabsorption syndrome. Curr Probl Radiol 1:3–47, 1971.

Masterson JB, Sweeney EC: The role of small bowel follow-through examination in the diagnosis of coeliac disease. Br J Radiol 49:660–664, 1976.

Olmsted WW, Reagin DE: Pathophysiology of enlargement of the small bowel fold. Am J Roentgenol 127:423–428, 1976.

Pepper HW, Brandborg LL, Shanser JD, Goldberg HI, Moss AA: Collagenous sprue. Am J Roentgenol 121:275–282, 1974.

Miscellaneous

Clemett AR, Marshak RH: Whipple's disease. Roentgen features and differential diagnosis. Radiol Clin North Am 7:105, 1969.

Davis TJ, Berk RN: Immunoglobulin deficiency diseases of the intestine. Gastrointest Radiol 2:7–11, 1977.

Legge DA, Carlson HC, Wollaeger EE: Roentgenologic appearance of systemic amyloidosis involving gastrointestinal tract. Am J Roentgenol 110:406–412, 1970.

Marshak RH, Hazzi C, Lindner AE, Maklansky D: Small bowel in immunoglobulin deficiency syndromes. Am J Roentgenol 122:227–240, 1974.

Marshak RH, Lindner AE, Maklansky D: Immunoglobulin disorders of the small bowel. Radiol Clin North Am 14:477–492, 1976.

Philips RL, Carlson HC: The roentgenographic and clinical findings in Whipple's disease. Am J Roentgenol 123:268–273, 1975.

9

VASCULAR DISEASE

Vascular disease is common in Western society. People tend to think of it in terms of ravaging effects of the heart, brain, and extremities. Vascular disease of the gut is often overlooked, usually to the patient's detriment. The disease can be insidious, but its manifestations run the gamut from mild diarrhea to florid bowel infarction and death of the patient.

ANATOMY OF CIRCULATION TO THE BOWEL

Consideration of this vitally important but consistently underrated topic will begin with a brief review of the blood supply to the bowel (Fig. 9–1). As illustrated in this figure, the superior mesenteric artery supplies the small bowel, the right colon, and the proximal

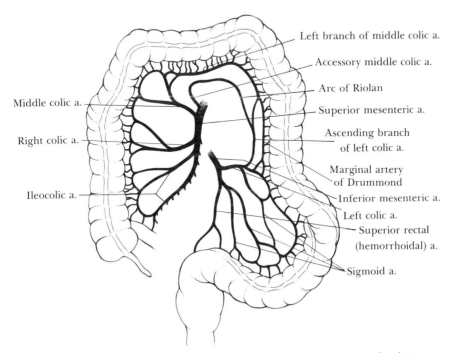

Figure 9–1. *Arterial supply to the colon.* Note anastomoses between superior and inferior mesenteric circulations.

147

and midtransverse colon. The inferior mesenteric artery supplies the left colon. Several facts emerge from a detailed examination of blood flow. The hallmark of intestinal blood flow is anastomosis; numerous anastomoses occur not only between branches of different arteries but also between branches of the same artery. These innumerable vessels form the so-called arcades or vasa recta of the bowel. The small bowel thus is particularly well vascularized, as is most of the colon; the rectosigmoid is likewise especially well vascularized because of myriad anastomoses. The splenic flexure region, on the other hand, is at risk because it lies in the so-called watershed area,* relying on anastomoses between the superior and inferior mesenteric arteries for adequate perfusion. As Meyers has shown, many people are at risk of developing ischemia of the splenic flexure because they lack adequate anastomoses between the two circulations.

In view of the apparently abundant blood supply to the gut, one might wonder how it could ever become ischemic. Occlusion of one or more major vessels by atheroma might go unnoticed if there is a good collateral blood supply. Of course, the more severe the atheroma, the easier it is to produce occlusion; thus, an acute embolus or thrombosis in one vessel might not be compensated for, and its end organ could become ischemic. It is also possible to imagine a subacute or chronic form of this process: vessels would gradually become narrower over a period of years, and at some point demand would outstrip supply.

MECHANISM OF ISCHEMIA

Not too many years ago the postulated mechanism for all cases of ischemia was *large vessel disease*, with a vessel being occluded by either atherosclerosis, thrombosis, or embolism. If collaterals were inadequate, the bowel supplied by the occluded vessel became ischemic. Over the past several decades, however, a new concept has been advanced by Boley and others, suggesting that a significant pro-

portion of intestinal ischemia is nonocclusive and is due instead to a *low-flow state*. In fact, this nonocclusive form of ischemia is being recognized more and more frequently, and accounts for over half the cases in many series.

In the low-flow state (which may be due to cardiac failure, hypovolemia, dehydration, shock, and so forth), mesenteric blood flow is temporarily reduced, precipitating an intense splanchnic vasoconstriction, which can persist long after what may have been a brief reduction in blood flow. It is this *persistent* splanchnic vasoconstriction that does the damage. *Let no one doubt just how devastating this disease can be: three of four patients will die.*

Boley and co-workers argue that aggressive diagnosis and treatment of ischemic disease can improve survival; they stress that *early recognition* is essential for successful treatment. Acute mesenteric ischemia usually occurs in an already ill patient: the one who has had a recent myocardial infarction or recent cardiac failure, one who has arrhythmias, or one in shock for any reason. Obviously, in a patient with valvular heart disease, an arrhythmia, or a recent myocardial infarction with mural thrombus, an embolus is also likely as the cause.

The precise etiology is important for *treatment* but *not for diagnosis.* Boley and colleagues stress the importance of a high index of suspicion: *"Any patient in the above [previously mentioned] categories who suddenly presents with abdominal pain, distention, or rectal bleeding should be suspected of having intestinal ischemia until proven otherwise."*

In attempting to make the diagnosis of ischemia, plain films of the abdomen should not be omitted; they can give important information. The cause of the abdominal catastrophe may be obvious, such as free intraperitoneal air. However, it should be stressed that, more often than not, in ischemia the plain films are *deceptively and disappointingly normal.* Nonspecific, localized ileus or a gasless abdomen may be the only clue.

As ischemia progresses to frank necrosis, the plain film may still remain negative, or findings may become less subtle (Fig. 9–2); at this stage, however, the patient's chances of survival also decrease. The bowel wall be-

---

*To understand this concept better, the dictionary defines a watershed as a ridge of high land dividing two areas that are drained by different river systems.

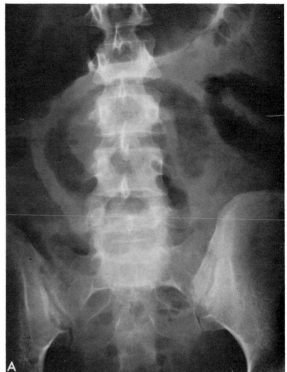

Figure 9–2. *Ischemic small bowel. A,* A plain film shows a number of abnormal loops of small bowel in the midabdomen with narrowing of the lumen, thickening of the wall, and effacement of the normal mucosal folds. The patient was taking contraceptive pills.

B, On small bowel follow-through to assess extent of disease, this is how it appears with contrast. There is marked thickening of the small bowel folds with "pinky-printing," characteristic of edema or blood in the submucosa, and separation of bowel loops due to thickening of the wall. Proximal to the ischemic area the bowel is dilated owing to partial obstruction.

C, A follow-up small bowel follow-through performed 10 days later shows almost complete resolution; this rapid reversal is characteristic of vascular disease.

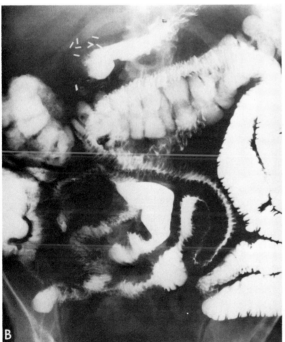

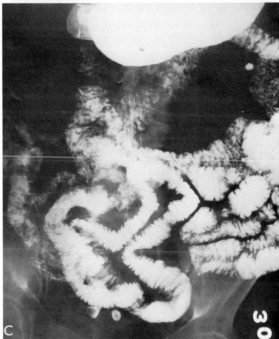

comes irregularly thickened owing to submucosal edema and hemorrhage; the small bowel loops will thus become separated from each other, as a result not only of thickened walls, but also of ascites. The folds become thickened and the intestinal contour becomes scalloped, resulting in "thumb-printing" in the colon and "pinky-printing" in the small bowel. The etiology is the same: submucosal edema and hemorrhage.

Eventually the small bowel lumen will become narrowed and featureless, the loops fixed and rigid. Gas may appear in the wall of the bowel, indicating gangrene and potential perforation. Gas in the portal vein is a very late and frequently preterminal sign, meaning that the bowel wall is definitely gangrenous; at this stage, the chance of survival is almost zero.

INTERVENTIONAL STUDIES

Obviously, angiography is the preferred way to study patients suspected of having ischemia. In practice, however, since ischemia is frequently not considered, or because it mimics other diseases, a barium study might be ordered and performed before angiography. The most significant finding on barium study is evidence of submucosal edema and hemorrhage: thickened folds, thumbprinting, separation of loops, narrowing of the lumen, and occasionally even evidence of mu-

cosal ulceration. In the colon, thumb-printing is most common (Fig. 9–3), but "transverse ridging" due to more diffuse intramural involvement and even fine ulcerations have been reported by Wittenberg. A cardinal feature of the barium findings in ischemic disease is that they change rapidly over time, and follow-up studies within 5 to 7 days will show this change.

What happens to the bowel depends on the severity of the ischemia. Marked ischemia leads to gangrene and its complications, but with milder ischemia, the bowel may return completely to normal. Thumb-printing will usually resolve within a few days as blood and edema resorb. However, the bowel may ulcerate or even perforate; then the involved area may heal by forming a stricture. It must be stressed again that bowel usually does return to normal following a *transient* ischemic episode.

Angiography is the study of choice if ischemia is suspected, because it can be both diagnostic and therapeutic. If angiography is

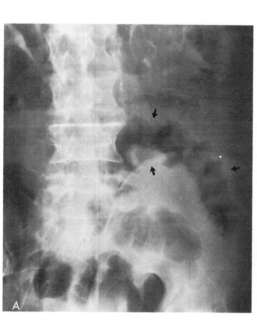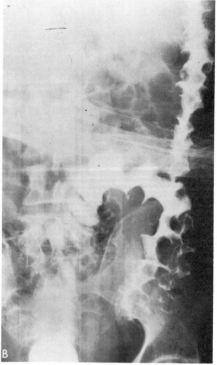

Figure 9–3. *Ischemic colitis. A,* On a plain abdominal film an abnormal loop of bowel is seen in the left midabdomen; the abnormality consists of soft tissue indentations (thumb-printing) (arrows). *B,* A barium enema confirms the presence of thumb-printing and shows disease extending from the sigmoid colon to the splenic flexure. The remainder of the colon was normal.

performed before actual infarction has taken place, and if the documented ischemia is vigorously treated with a vasodilator such as papaverine, an appreciable improvement in survival is possible.

So far the discussion has been about acute *arterial* disease. *Venous* compromise can also occur and result in infarction. There is also a chronic form of arterial disease, chronic mesenteric ischemia, sometimes called "intestinal angina." Patients with this disorder classically present with abdominal pain shortly after eating. In most of these patients, atherosclerotic narrowing of vessels is the proposed etiology, although precise standards for diagnosis and treatment are controversial.

SMALL VESSEL DISEASE

Not all ischemic disease can or should be attributed to the larger vessels. "Small vessel disease" includes an interesting assortment of conditions with which radiologists should be familiar.

Inflammatory Disease

Inflammatory vascular disease, or vasculitis, may be either primary or due to some other disease. Among the causes of primary vasculitis are periarteritis nodosa, systemic lupus erythematosus, and other collagen disorders. Secondary arteritis can occur after radiation or as part of inflammatory bowel disease. Diabetes may affect either large or small vessels. In any of these small vessel diseases, the same spectrum from mild mucosal abnormalities to full-thickness infarction can occur, but the changes will tend to be patchy rather than confined to a specific vascular distribution.

Noninflammatory Disease

Noninflammatory small vessel abnormalities also encompass some interesting lesions, such as vascular malformations. These can occur anywhere and may bleed, but they can be extremely difficult to diagnose. Angiodysplasia, especially in the right colon, has been associated with aortic stenosis. These small vessel abnormalities are best diagnosed by angiography, although even angiography fails to detect many small vascular malformations.

Effect of Drugs

No discussion of ischemic bowel disease would be complete without mention of the effect of many drugs on blood flow to the gut. Some very commonly used drugs, such as digitalis, can constrict the splanchnic circulation and exacerbate a low-flow state. Oral contraceptives are known to have thromboembolic complications, and the gut is not spared; both arterial and venous thrombotic disease has been associated with "the pill."

OTHER VASCULAR PROBLEMS

Varices

Varices are important vascular lesions with which every radiologist must be familiar. These represent collateral venous channels that open up when blood flow from the bowel to the liver via splenic, mesenteric, or portal veins is impeded. In Western society, these are most commonly due to cirrhosis of the liver. Any age group can present with varices, which are most common and most easily demonstrated around the esophagus; gastric and duodenal varices are also reasonably common but less easy to demonstrate. Varices can be studied by barium swallow, esophagoscopy, or angiography. Small varices begin as mild thickening and tortuosity of the normally thin parallel folds of the esophagus and progress to large, serpiginous, wormlike structures that distort the normal fold pattern and cause scalloping of the esophageal contour (Fig. 9–4). Several methods have been advocated to look for varices using a dense barium preparation and filming in the supine position; the films are taken in gentle suspended respiration. The aim is to have a relaxed esophagus coated with barium so that the fold pattern can be optimally seen. A distended, barium-filled esophagus will not demonstrate small varices

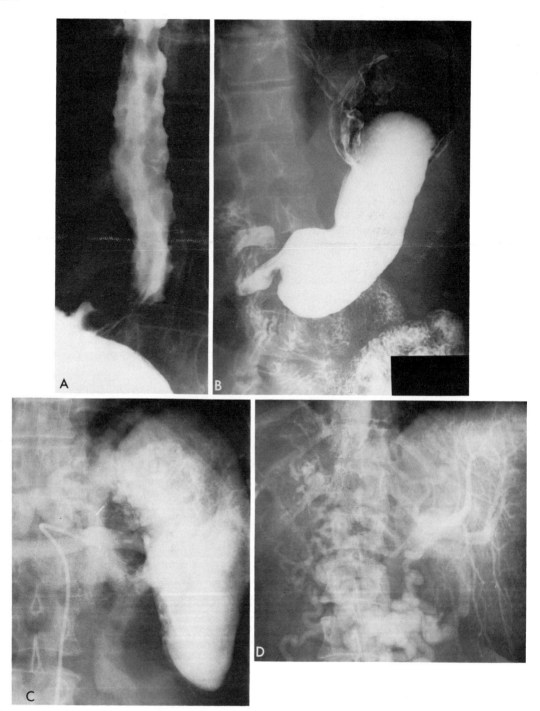

Figure 9–4. *A, Esophageal varices.* Barium swallow shows multiple serpiginous filling defects in the distal esophagus. Note the scalloped contour of the edge of the esophagus when the varices are profiled.

B, Gastric varices. Multiple irregular filling defects are seen within the fundus of the stomach concentrated around the gastroesophageal junction. There is also slight irregularity of the folds in the distal esophagus, indicating esophageal varices.

C, Angiogram, venous phase, corresponding to the upper GI series in *B.* Note the large multiple tortuous veins corresponding to the filling defects seen in *B.*

D, Another angiogram demonstrating that varices can occur anywhere within the abdomen and not just around the gastroesophageal junction.

because they will be completely collapsed by overdistention. It should again be stressed that varices will not necessarily be demonstrable on every swallow in every projection. As the veins fill and collapse, they will alternately be demonstrable and disappear during barium examination.

The varices described here are called *uphill* varices because blood tries to *ascend* around the block in the liver to reach the heart. *Downhill* varices also occur. These form when blood from the upper body attempts to descend to the heart, via venous collaterals, around a blocked superior vena cava. The vena cava is most commonly blocked by pressure from an adjacent mediastinal tumor, resulting in the acute superior vena cava syndrome. These downhill varices about the upper esophagus can also be demonstrated on barium swallow.

Hemorrhage and Hematoma

Finally, *hemorrhage* into the wall of the bowel will also be included under the broad umbrella of "vascular" disease. Hemorrhage can occur as the result of drugs (anticoagulants), trauma, or a bleeding diathesis. Classically, the bowel lesion is localized to a relatively short segment. The blood is in the submucosa, resulting in fold thickening and a "picketfence" or stack-of-coins appearance; there may also be pinky-printing. As in other processes that involve the wall, the lumen is slightly narrowed, and the loop separated from its neighbors assumes a hammock-like configuration.

A more sharply localized hemorrhage (hematoma) is a frequent occurrence in the duodenal region (Fig. 9–5), seen commonly in young people after blunt abdominal trauma. This relatively fixed segment takes the brunt of the trauma for two reasons; because it is retroperitoneal, it is fixed in position, and with trauma it is compressed against the spine. Localized bleeding of this type can cause duodenal obstruction, but treatment is usually conservative because the hematoma resolves by itself; occasionally surgical evacuation is necessary.

In summary, vascular disease involving the gastrointestinal tract takes many forms, some serious, some not. Mild, reversible dis-

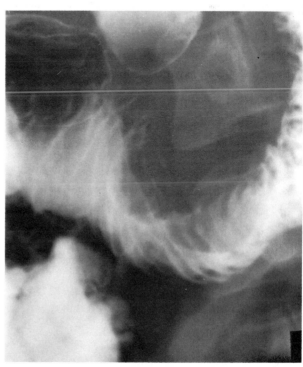

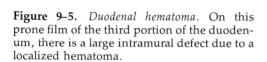

Figure 9–5. *Duodenal hematoma.* On this prone film of the third portion of the duodenum, there is a large intramural defect due to a localized hematoma.

ease (for example, some cases of ischemic colitis) is probably underdiagnosed. The full-blown picture of ischemia has a very poor prognosis, with a mortality rate well over 50 per cent. This is particularly true of ischemia of the small bowel; ischemic colitis tends to have a more benign course. Those who advocate an aggressive diagnostic and therapeutic approach have shown that this can make a significant improvement in survival. The key is to consider the possibility of ischemia in any patient with the acute onset of unexplained abdominal pain and bleeding from the GI tract.

References

General

Boley SJ, Schwartz SS, Williams LF: Vascular Disorders of the Intestine. New York, Appleton-Century-Crofts, 1971.
Schwartz S, Boley SJ, Robinson K, Krieger H, Schultz L, Allen AC: Roentgenologic features of vascular disorders of the intestines. Radiol Clin North Am 2:71–87, 1964.
Wang CC, Reeves JD: Mesenteric vascular disease. Am J Roentgenol 83:895–908, 1960.

Interventional Studies

Athanasoulis CA: Therapeutic applications of angiography (first of two parts). N Engl J Med 302:1117–1179, 1980.
Boley SJ, Sprayregan S, Siegelman SS, Veith FJ: Initial results from an aggressive roentgenological and surgical approach to acute mesenteric ischemia. Surgery 81:848–855, 1977.
Johnsrude IS, Jackson DC: The role of the radiologist in acute gastrointestinal bleeding. Gastrointest Radiol 3:357, 1978.
Pond GD, Ovitt TW: Therapeutic applications of angiography: state of the art. Curr Probl Diagn Radiol 9:3, 1979.

Sheedy PF II, Fulton RE, Atwell DT: Angiographic evaluation of patients with chronic gastrointestinal bleeding. Am J Roentgenol 123:338, 1975.
Wittenberg J, Athanasoulis CA, Shapiro JH, Williams LF Jr: A radiological approach to the patient with acute, extensive bowel ischemia. Radiology 106:13–24, 1973.

Small Bowel

Balthazar EJ, Einhorn R: Intramural gastrointestinal hemorrhage. Clinical and radiographic manifestations. Gastrointest Radiol 1:229–239, 1976.
Ghahremani GG, Meyers MA, Forman J, Port RB: Ischemic disease of the small bowel and colon associated with oral contraceptives. Gastrointest Radiol 2:221–228, 1977.
Joffe N, Goldman H, Antonioli DA: Barium studies in small-bowel infarction. Radiological-pathological correlation. Radiology 123:303–309, 1977.
Mellins HZ, Rigler LG: The roentgen findings in strangulating obstructions of the small intestine. Am J Roentgenol 71:404, 1954.
Wiot JF: Intramural small intestine hemorrhage — a differential diagnosis. Semin Roentgenol 1:219–233, 1966.

Colon

Eisenberg RL, Montgomery CK, Margulis AR: Colitis in the elderly: ischemic colitis mimicking ulcerative and granulomatous colitis. Am J Roetngenol 133:1113, 1979.
Meyers MA: Griffiths' point: Critical anastomosis at the splenic flexure. Significance in ischemia of the colon. Am J Roentgenol 126:1, 1977.
Whitehouse GH, Watt J: Ischemic colitis associated with carcinoma of the colon. Gastrointest Radiol 2:31–35, 1977.
Wittenberg J, Athanasoulis CA, Williams LF, Paredes S, O'Sullivan P, Brown B: Ischemic colitis: radiology and pathophysiology. Am J Roentgenol 123:287, 1975.

Varices

Cockerill EM, Miller RE, Chernish SM, McLaughlin GC, Rodda BE: Optimal visualization of esophageal varices. Am J Roentgenol 126:512–523, 1976.
Evans JA, Delany F: Gastric varices. Radiology 60:46–52, 1953.

10

THE POSTOPERATIVE PATIENT

Examination of the postoperative patient is a constant challenge to the gastrointestinal radiologist, especially the novice. Things happen quickly and in seemingly unpredictable fashion during these studies, which can confuse the unprepared examiner. This uncomfortable situation can be considerably defused by an understanding of the relevant surgical anatomy and the expected postoperative appearances.

If the saying "forewarned is forearmed" has any validity in GI radiology, it is in the examination of the postoperative patient. It is crucial to know that a patient has had surgery *before* beginning the examination. A good habit to get into is always to ask the patient before beginning whether he has had surgery, since in many cases this crucial information will not be provided (sometimes the clinician himself may not know). It is vital for the radiologist to know whether the examination will be on a postoperative GI tract before "spilling the first drop of barium" for two reasons: it will influence (1) *what* study to perform and (2) *how* to perform that study, i.e., how much of what density contrast medium is used, what position is used initially, and so forth.

BASELINE STUDY

One very important and helpful aid is a previous postoperative study for comparison;

this will help in interpreting the unfamiliar anatomy and radiographic appearance. Ideally, all postoperative patients should have a *baseline study* performed within the first few months of surgery, to define the altered anatomy and changes due to scarring. As will be discussed, this is of inestimable value in diagnosing recurrent disease.

There are several important reasons for follow-up studies in the postoperative patient. In the immediate postoperative period, it may become clinically obvious that the patient is not responding appropriately. A study may then be requested to search for *early* complications, such as a leak, or obstruction at the anastomosis, which may be due to edema or technical error. As time passes, *late* complications are more likely to be seen, such as strictures or recurrent disease.

A wide range of surgery on the GI tract will now be discussed, with comments on radiologic techniques and diagnosis. For this discussion a strictly anatomic approach seems most convenient.

ESOPHAGUS

Surgery on the *esophagus* can be performed for benign or malignant disease. "Benign" disease would include diverticula, strictures, hernias, and so forth. When a Zenker's diverticulum is resected, the esophagus must be sutured closed at the resection site, and a

155

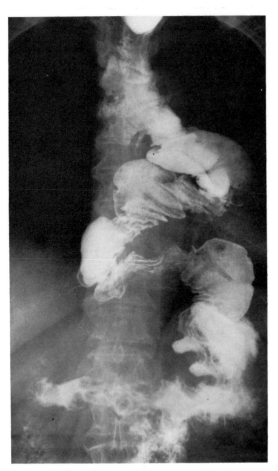

Figure 10–1. *Esophageal replacement (colon interposition).* The colon has been swung up into the chest as a conduit. The usual location is substernal, although either subcutaneous or posterior placement is an option.

leak or stricture at the site can occur. Resection of a stricture may involve a local resection and reanastomosis or, for more extensive strictures, esophageal bypass. Colon is usually the replacement organ and the appearance of a colonic interposition is characteristic (Fig. 10–1); small bowel may also be used.

Surgery for malignant disease similarly involves either bypass or resection and reanastomosis. Removal of tumor-containing esophagus, along with a portion of stomach, and esophagogastric anastomosis is such an example. Unfortunately, the surgical treatment of esophageal carcinoma is not very successful, and recurrence is common; distal tumors are easier to resect technically and have a better prognosis.

HIATUS HERNIA REPAIR

Repair of a hiatus hernia can be accomplished in a number of ways. One of the most common operations is the *Nissen fundoplication,* the characteristic radiographic appearance of which might be mistaken for disease by the unwary (Fig. 10–2). The Nissen repair involves reducing the hernia and wrapping the fundus of the stomach around the reduced esophagus to create an antireflux mechanism. Following successful surgery, a hernia should no longer be demonstrable, there should be no reflux, and a characteristic "pseudotumor" will be seen in the fundus. This fundic filling defect, caused by tissue wrapped around the distal esophagus, can easily be mistaken for a neoplasm, if a history of surgery is not available. Incidentally, the wrap can be made too tight, in which case the patient suffers from an iatrogenic esophageal obstruction; conversely, if it is too loose, the patient will continue to reflux, another failure.

Examinations performed within the first few days of esophageal surgery are usually done looking for a leak at the anastomotic site, or to confirm that all is well before the patient begins eating again. These examinations are usually performed with a water-soluble contrast medium unless a tracheoesophageal fistula is suspected, in which case it would be harmful to use water-soluble contrast. If no leak is demonstrated, then barium may be used to define the anatomy more clearly. In addition to leaks, anastomotic obstruction can be excluded at this time.

STOMACH

Many operations can be performed on the stomach, most of which involve the resection of varying amounts of stomach with subsequent reanastomosis; anatomic continuity may be reestablished or the anatomy may be altered.

Those cases in which anatomic continuity is reestablished (gastroduodenostomy) are known as Billroth I (BI) operations; those with altered anatomy (gastroenterostomy) are loosely grouped together as Billroth II (BII)

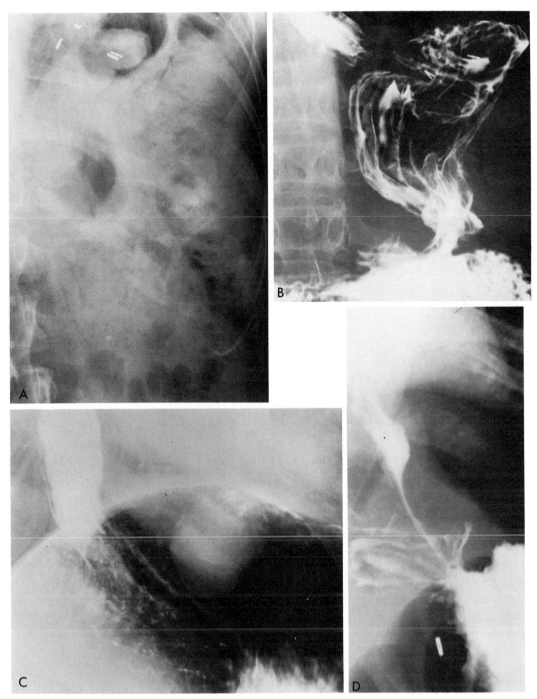

Figure 10–2. *Nissen fundoplication. A, On the plain film* clips are seen near the gastroesophageal junction. There is a large soft tissue mass projecting into the gastric fundus, which could be mistaken for a tumor. *B,* Following barium administration, this pseudotumor is delineated. Compare the pseudotumor with the soft tissue mass in *C,* which is remote from the gastroesophageal junction and was a leiomyoma. *D,* One of the complications of the Nissen procedure is shown: marked narrowing of the distal esophagus due to too tight a wrap.

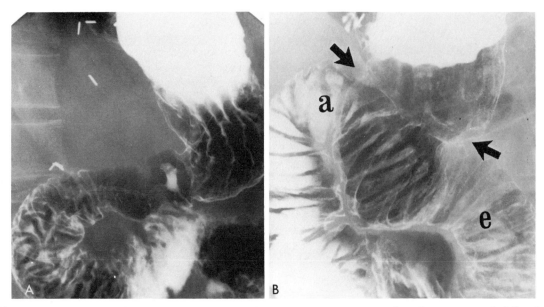

Figure 10–3. *A, Billroth I anastomosis.* Note that anatomic continuity has been restored following antrectomy and vagotomy with reanastomosis of the duodenum to the stomach. Incidentally, the pool of barium at the anastomosis represented a recurrent ulcer.

B, Billroth II anastomosis. The anastomotic line is well demonstrated (arrows) and there is equal filling of both the afferent *(a)* and efferent *(e)* loops. Good distention and coating have been obtained of both the anastomosis and the loops.

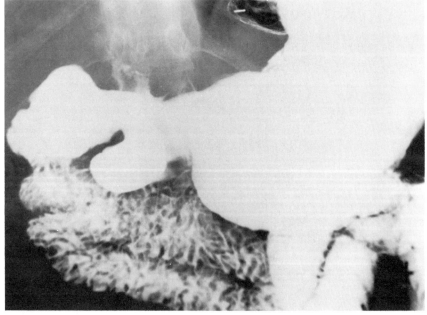

Figure 10–4. *Pyloroplasty.* There is marked deformity in the region of the pylorus and the normally narrow pyloric canal is now wide open. A large, rounded "beagle-ear" deformity is seen on the greater curvature; on the lesser curvature another projection is seen. Both of these would be compatible with surgical change but in fact the one on the lesser curvature was an acute ulcer. This illustrates the problem of diagnosing ulceration in the presence of surgical deformity.

(Fig. 10–3). In a BII anastomosis, a jejunal loop is brought up to the greater curvature; this is the *efferent* loop. The duodenal stump is closed off and becomes part of the *afferent* loop. A little review of Latin helps clarify the names of these loops: the efferent loop (i.e., *ex* = away from or out of) drains away from the stomach distally; the afferent loop (*a* from *ad* = toward) leads from the duodenum to the stomach and drains bile and pancreatic secretions from this "blind loop."

Surgery for peptic ulcer disease has gone through many cycles, and many different procedures have been claimed as the "ideal" treatment. Two common procedures are antrectomy, and pyloroplasty and vagotomy (P and V), both procedures being designed to decrease gastric acid output. As a vagotomy results in delayed gastric emptying, a concomitant drainage procedure is necessary (pyloroplasty). The pyloroplasty results in a characteristic appearance, which should not be confused with disease (Fig. 10–4); incidentally, finding an ulcer after a pyloroplasty can be very difficult owing to the presence of this surgical deformity.

As already stated, it is important to know before beginning the examination that the study will be on a postoperative stomach. A judicious amount of contrast medium must be used, so that the anatomy can be clearly defined without flooding the gastric remnant with barium and completely obscuring both it and the anastomosis: no more than a few ounces of contrast should be given initially. The flow of the contrast must be observed fluoroscopically right from the beginning so that the anatomy can be determined and the patient positioned properly for subsequent films.

Since normal anatomic continuity is preserved in a Billroth I, the patient can be positioned as usual to obtain stomach and duodenal sweep views; positioning a patient with Billroth II for maximum advantage can be more difficult. The initial swallow should pinpoint the remnant, the anastomosis, and the efferent and afferent loops. Since what is done at surgery varies even with the "standard" operation, not every patient can be studied precisely the same way. It is helpful, however, to have the patient supine and usually somewhat turned onto the right side to visualize the anastomosis best. Sometimes placing the patient in an oblique position in the opposite direction (left side to table) will display the anatomy better. Keeping the patient semisupine and initially using only small sips of contrast medium will prevent too much fluid from flooding jejunal loops and obscuring the crucial anastomotic area. Once the anatomy is clear evaluation of the anastomosis can begin. Is it patent or is there an anatomic cause for outlet obstruction, such as postoperative edema, which can severely limit the anastomotic lumen? A technical error can create an anastomosis that is too small and which impedes gastric emptying (Fig. 10–5). In the *immediate* postoperative period, the examination can often be limited to the region of the anastomosis.

Recurrent disease, either neoplastic or inflammatory, also commonly involves the anastomosis. Ulcers can recur at the anastomosis, but it should be pointed out that the term "anastomotic ulcer" is somewhat of a misnomer; most recurrent ulcers following gastrojejunostomy are actually in the *efferent loop* (Fig. 10–6), within a few centimeters of the anastomosis. This is why it is so critical to study both the anastomosis and the proximal efferent limb carefully at the beginning of the examination; significant pathology will be missed if barium has flooded the small bowel and obscured these areas.

As it is, the routine examination of the postoperative stomach is notoriously inaccurate; only about half of proven anastomotic ulcers are actually found on routine examination. There are a number of reasons for this inaccuracy, including the already alluded to "flooding" with too much contrast medium. Another reason is that it can be extremely difficult to keep the remnant and anastomosis distended; compression is of little value because the remnant is high up, under the ribs. There are probably as many false positives as false negatives; one of the commonest is to mistake a pseudodiverticulum resulting from surgery for an ulcer.

For these reasons, many advocate primary double contrast examination of the postopera-

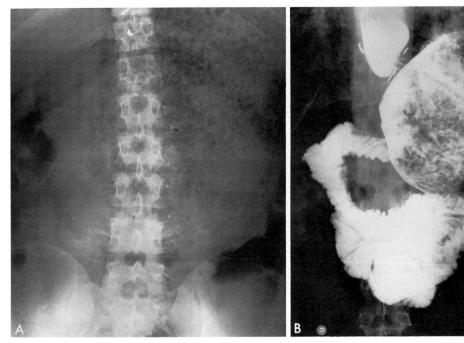

Figure 10–5. *Anastomotic narrowing with bezoar. A,* Mottled densities are apparent in the left upper quadrant of the abdomen, making one suspect an abscess or an ischemic loop, but because it is in the expected location of the stomach, a stomach full of debris must be excluded. Note that the transverse colon is displaced downwards. *B,* A barium study was therefore performed, demonstrating that this appearance was due to semisolid and solid conglomerate of food and vegetable matter (a bezoar). This may be a result of either functional or organic outlet obstruction.

tive stomach. A thick barium preparation, a large amount of gas, and a large dose of glucagon (0.5 to 1.0 mg) are necessary for success. Note should be made that, in the postoperative patient, there is no longer a "sphincter" (pylorus) to retain air and barium for a leisurely study, so a speedy examination is especially important.

Following a careful examination of the anastomosis and efferent loop, additional

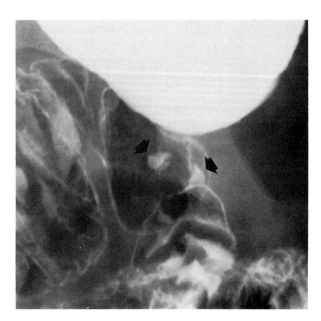

Figure 10–6. *Recurrent ulceration following Billroth II operation.* Within the proximal efferent loop are two collections of barium (arrows), representing acute ulcers. Note that often, with these ulcers, radiating folds cannot be demonstrated.

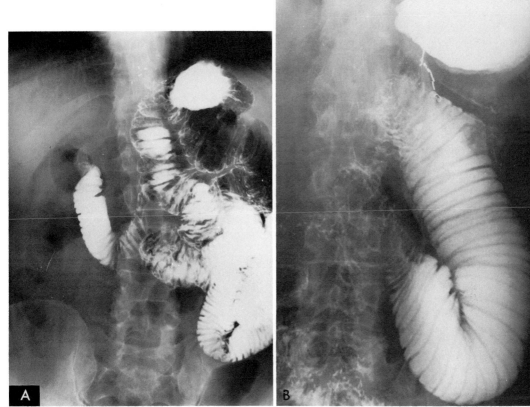

Figure 10–7. *Normal Billroth II anastomosis with demonstration of afferent loop. A,* The duodenal stump and descending portion of the duodenum are filled with contrast medium and appear normal in size. *B, Afferent loop obstruction;* compare this with appearance in *A.* The afferent loop has become progressively more dilated and fails to empty in the normal fashion.

barium and air are given to distend the gastric remnant so it can be examined fully. The efferent loop should fill by gravity, without positional manipulation, unless it is obstructed. The afferent loop is more difficult to fill, and sometimes it is necessary to turn the patient onto his right side to fill it; sometimes compression over the efferent loop helps to fill the afferent loop. It is as important to study the afferent loop as it is the efferent. The afferent loop can become functionally obstructed *(afferent loop syndrome)* (Fig. 10–7), resulting in significant morbidity. As much as possible of the afferent loop should be filled to ensure that an adequate gastric resection has been performed. Occasionally, some antrum is inadvertently left behind *(retained antrum),* and when this can be documented, it becomes obvious why the patient's ulcer diathesis persists.

Carcinoma in the Postoperative Stomach

Careful examination of the gastric remnant is essential regardless of why the initial surgery was performed. If the original operation was for cancer, recurrent disease would not be unexpected. Be aware, however, that there is also an increased risk of developing cancer in the gastric remnant (Fig. 10–8), *even if the original surgery was for benign disease.* Beyond 15 years after surgery, the risk of developing cancer in the gastric remnant increases rapidly so that by 25 years after operation, the risk is some six times that of the general population. Careful examination of the remnant, ideally with the double contrast method, is obviously essential; any indistensible areas should be immediately suspected of being cancerous.

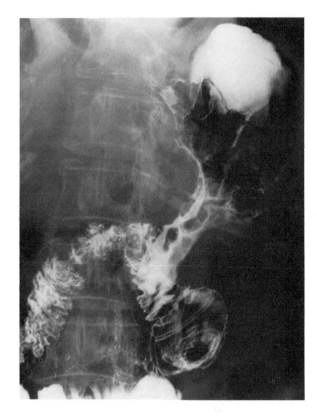

Figure 10–8. *Carcinoma following Billroth II anastomosis.* Narrowing, rigidity, and deformity of the distal recurrent anastomosis and proximal efferent loop are seen. The folds in this region are thickened and irregular owing to infiltration by tumor.

One other condition occasionally affects the gastric remnant: retrograde jejunal intussusception. In this condition, there will be a gastric filling defect with a "coiled-spring" pattern; this intussusception can cause outlet obstruction.

Examination of the postoperative stomach is obviously somewhat more complicated than usual and demands a special approach. Try not to get into the predicament of having a remnant and small bowel so full of barium that detailed examination of critical areas is impossible. This can be avoided if (1) the patient is known to have had gastric surgery, (2) the type of surgery is known, and (3) the examination is tailored to suit the patient's particular circumstances.

COLON

The postoperative appearance of the upper gastrointestinal tract is familiar to most radiologists. Less emphasis, however, has been placed on the appearance of the postoperative colon. It is incumbent upon radiologists to master this subject as thoroughly as that of the upper tract. Most of the same principles apply; the difference is merely in anatomy and terminology.

As with the upper tract, the major difficulty in studying the postoperative colon is to distinguish postsurgical change from recurrent disease. The radiologist must become familiar with a wide variety of normal postoperative appearances and must be able to identify that critical area, the anastomosis, where recurrent disease is most likely to occur.

Numerous operations have been devised for a variety of colonic diseases, including polyps, cancer, inflammatory bowel disease, and diverticulitis. In some operations, such as the definitive treatment for ulcerative colitis, the whole colon is removed and ceases to be of concern to the radiologist. (Even if a tiny sleeve of rectum is left, follow-up is almost invariably by sigmoidoscopy rather than by barium examination.) Most colonic surgery, however, involves removing the diseased segment with enough colon remaining to necessitate reexamination at a later date. Follow-up studies are particularly important in patients who are at high risk for developing cancer: those whose first operation was for colonic cancer, those with multiple polyps, and those with pancolitis. Such follow-up studies are usually performed annually or semiannually.

Colonic surgery can be approached most simply by considering it in several major categories: (1) the diseased segment is removed and colonic continuity is reestablished; (2) the diseased segment is removed, but colonic continuity is not reestablished immediately; obviously in this case a concurrent diverting procedure must be performed; (3) colostomy alone can be performed without any colonic resection. Which type of procedure is performed depends on the underlying bowel disease, as well as the condition of the bowel and adjacent tissues at the time of surgery.

A colostomy may be either temporary or permanent. For example, it is common to perform a colostomy to rest the distal colon following resection for acute diverticulitis. Before the colostomy can be closed, the radiologist will be asked to evaluate the integrity and patency of the anastomosis. If a permanent colostomy is necessary for an inoperable distal carcinoma, the radiologist will be asked to evaluate the proximal colon via the colostomy for concurrent or recurrent disease.

Before considering the different types of anastomoses in detail, the options the surgeon has when operating on the colon will be examined. The major decision the surgeon must make is whether to perform a resection and primary anastomosis or whether to divert the colon (diverting colostomy) and consider secondary reanastomosis at a later time. This is a clinical decision based on the disease process and the general condition of the patient.

The surgical therapy for diverticulitis is somewhat controversial. Several stages and multiple operations are frequently necessary in the treatment of this disease. Occasionally surgeons advocate primary repair: the diseased segment is resected and the colon is reanastomosed in continuity; this is seldom possible in the acutely ill patient. Most believe that the inflammatory reaction jeopardizes the anastomosis and counsel a two-stage or even three-stage repair. A diverting colostomy is an integral part of this procedure; the distal bowel is "rested" and protected from the fecal stream. Decompressive, protective operations are also helpful when bowel integrity is questioned for any other reason and breakdown of the anastomosis could occur. An example is obstruction, when the bowel has been grossly dilated.

Surgery for rectal lesions depends on the location of the tumor. Lesions well above the posterior peritoneal reflection can be handled with anterior resection and primary anastomosis. On the other hand, resection of a very *low* rectal lesion (at or below 5.5 cm in women and 7 cm in men from the anal verge) would not leave enough rectal tissue to permit a safe and continent reanastomosis. An abdominoperineal operation (*Miles* operation) is necessary, and the patient must have a permanent colostomy.

Types of Anastomosis. There are three basic ways to reanastomose the colon after resection: (1) end-to-end, (2) end-to-side, (3) side-to-side (Fig. 10–9). Each has advantages and disadvantages suitable for specific types of colon surgery, as will be discussed.

The end-to-end anastomosis is commonly used for segmental resections and is the most physiologic anastomosis. It is particularly suitable when two segments of bowel have lumens of the same diameter — for example, in the sigmoid colon. End-to-side anastomoses can be performed in different parts of the colon. They are most frequently used for bypass with exclusion or when lumens are of disparate sizes (ileocolostomy or rectosigmoid anastomosis). Side-to-side anastomosis is the safest and least likely to leak, but is the least physiologic and prone to formation of blind loops and intussusception.

As in the stomach, the most critical region in the postoperative colon is the anastomosis. The majority of significant disease will occur at this site, either early in the postoperative course or months or years later. The radiologist must demonstrate this region adequately. Knowing what kind of surgery was done is an immense help, because the radiologist now

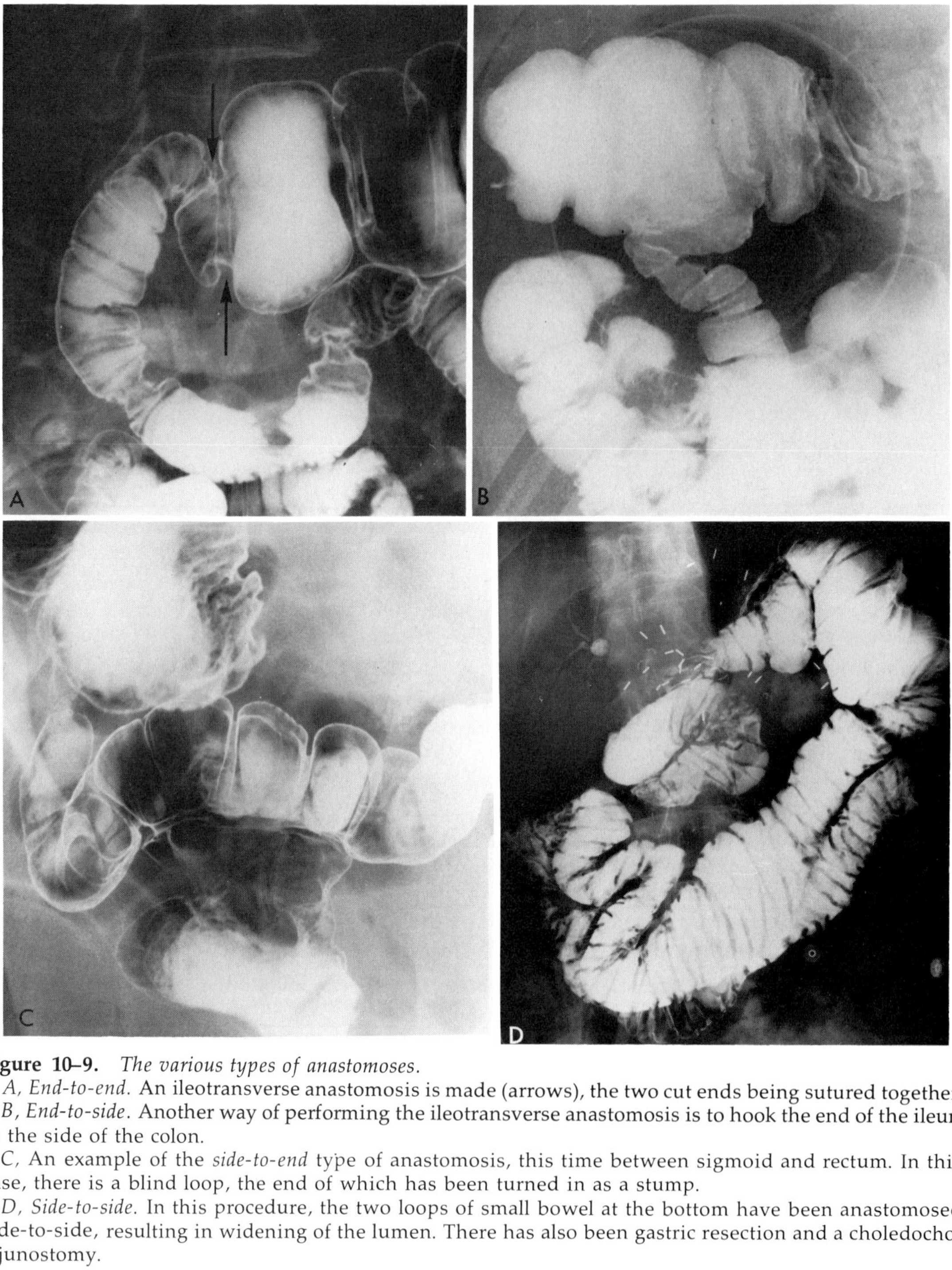

Figure 10–9. *The various types of anastomoses.*

A, End-to-end. An ileotransverse anastomosis is made (arrows), the two cut ends being sutured together.

B, End-to-side. Another way of performing the ileotransverse anastomosis is to hook the end of the ileum to the side of the colon.

C, An example of the *side-to-end* type of anastomosis, this time between sigmoid and rectum. In this case, there is a blind loop, the end of which has been turned in as a stump.

D, Side-to-side. In this procedure, the two loops of small bowel at the bottom have been anastomosed side-to-side, resulting in widening of the lumen. There has also been gastric resection and a choledocho-jejunostomy.

knows *where* to look for the anastomosis, which is certainly the first step in radiographing it adequately.

Immediate postoperative complications, as with any anastomosis, include anastomotic rupture (blow-out) (Fig. 10–10); these can be documented with water-soluble contrast medium. Careful fluoroscopy and technique are important. Gastrografin must be introduced slowly, under low pressure (low bag); care must be taken not to overdistend and thus overstress the operative area. The inflow of contrast medium must be stopped immediately if any extravasation is demonstrated.

There are several late complications with which the radiologist must be familiar. The most serious is recurrent disease (cancer or inflammatory bowel disease), usually at the anastomosis. Cancer recurs in over 10 per cent of cases, usually at the anastomosis; tumor

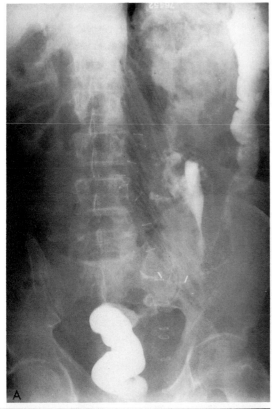

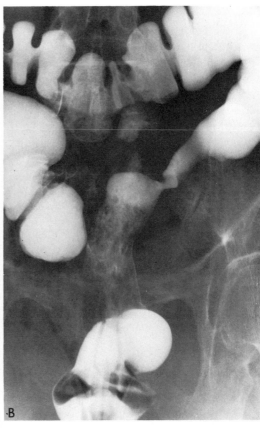

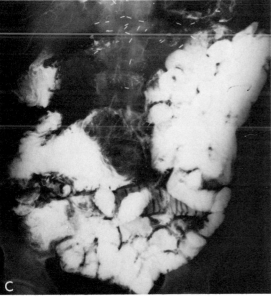

Figure 10–10. *Complications of the anastomosis (early and late).*

A, Ruptured anastomosis. Gastrografin enema shows a retroperitoneal rupture of a retroperitoneal colonic anastomosis. Note not only the extravasation of contrast material but also the streaky air due to dissection along the psoas muscle bundles.

B, Some months following colon anastomosis, a barium enema reveals marked narrowing at the anastomotic site, representing a *benign stricture.*

C, Another late complication is *intussusception,* and this is particularly common in the side-to-side anastomosis. This study is from the same patient as in Figure 10–9D, who had a side-to-side anastomosis in the proximal small bowel. Note the large filling defect within the dilated loop, representing an intussusception.

seeding at the time of surgery is postulated. Granulomatous disease recurs in up to 50 per cent of cases, usually on the small bowel side of the anastomosis.

Recurrent Disease

It is frequently difficult to distinguish postsurgical change from recurrent disease. Fleischner stresses that surgical changes are more likely to be circular, causing concentric filling defects. Recurrent cancer, especially if found early, presents as an eccentric filling defect (Fig. 10–11). Spasm and edema resulting from surgery can produce filling defects too, but these also tend to be concentric. A central tenet in the interpretation of the postoperative examination is comparison of it with a *baseline study*. This is of such importance that it must be stressed at the risk of being repetitive. This is the easiest way to differentiate between postsurgical defects and actual disease. Ideally, the baseline study should be performed within a few months of surgery; by this time the anastomosis will have healed but it will be too early for any radiographically apparent recurrent disease to appear. Surgical deformities will be documented on this early study; frequently changes caused by edema and spasm will also be seen. Edema and spasm should gradually subside, but anatomic

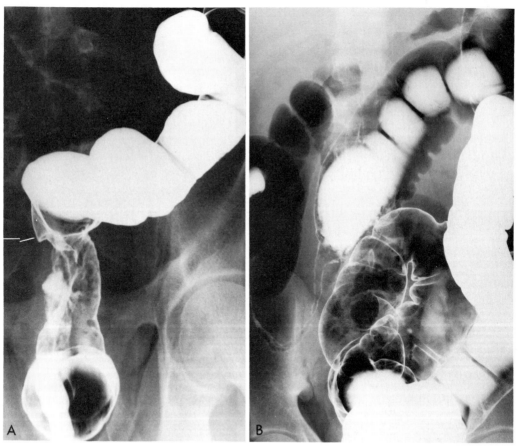

Figure 10–11. *Recurrent disease.*

A, Recurrent carcinoma. A rectosigmoid anastomosis with an irregular ulcerated mass is present on one wall of the rectum; this begins at the anastomosis and is extending distally. Note the proximal overhanging edge (arrow).

B, Recurrent Crohn's disease. On the small bowel side of an ileotransverse anastomosis, there is marked narrowing of the bowel lumen over a long segment. The small bowel is also dilated proximally owing to partial obstruction.

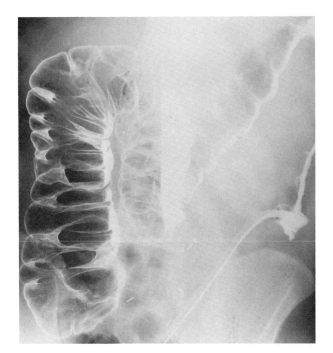

Figure 10–12. *Colostomy enema with double contrast.* A double contrast enema through the colostomy not only can be performed successfully, as illustrated here, but also is an excellent method to look for recurrent cancer.

defects may persist indefinitely. Obviously, any change, any newly identifiable lesion (especially one that is growing) documented subsequent to the baseline study must be considered recurrent disease until proved otherwise. Other types of infrequent lesions, such as a suture granuloma, have been reported, but most lesions, unfortunately, will be recurrent disease. *Detailed mucosal views of the anastomosis* are essential for complete evaluation; the double contrast method is particularly useful in the detailed examination of the mucosa necessary to document recurrent disease and is advocated as the primary method of examination.

The radiologist must be alert for more than just recurrent disease. A postoperative examination is essential for finding concurrent tumors; some 3 per cent of patients will present with a second primary tumor. A good double contrast examination is especially useful in demonstrating those polyps that are potentially malignant.

Patients with colostomies also require follow-up studies, but because these must be performed via the colostomy (Fig. 10–12) they are somewhat more difficult to do than routine postoperative enemas. In the patient with a temporary colostomy, radiologic studies are

directed at assessing the diverted colon prior to hook-up; these are usually done using single contrast. In the patient with a permanent colostomy, however, recurrent disease is being sought, and although previously single contrast was used, the double contrast method may now be preferable.

Ureterosigmoidostomy

A special type of colonic anastomosis that is occasionally performed and has a characteristic appearance not easily confused with other anastomoses is the ureterosigmoidostomy, performed as a urinary diversion procedure (Fig. 10–13). Follow-up studies are particularly important after this anastomosis, because there is increased risk of developing colonic carcinoma, presumably as a result of urinary metabolites bathing the colonic mucosa.

Appendectomy

Finally, one important nonanastomotic postoperative change in the colon should be mentioned — the appendectomy defect (Fig. 10–14). This is a filling defect along the *medial*

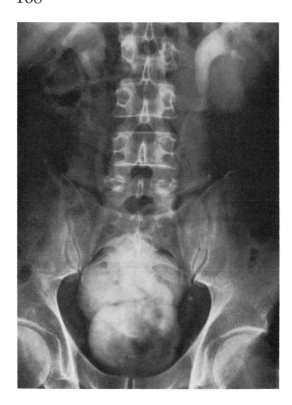

Figure 10–13. *Ureterosigmoidostomy.* This film from an intravenous urogram shows the ureters entering the sigmoid loop. Any filling defects within this loop should raise the question of a polyp or carcinoma.

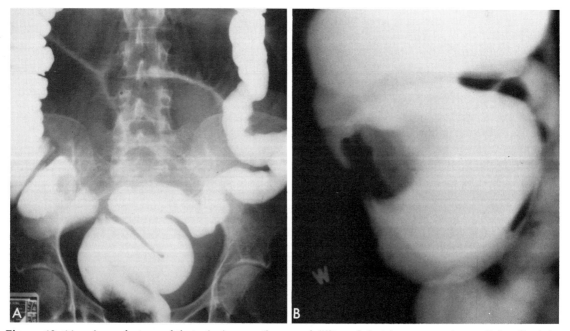

Figure 10–14. *Appendectomy defect. A,* A smooth, round filling defect is seen on the *medial* wall of the cecum. Compare this with *B,* in which there is an irregular lobulated defect on the *lateral* wall; the latter was a carcinoma.

wall of the cecum caused by the invaginated appendiceal stump. This defect should not be confused with a tumor. Obviously, a history of previous appendectomy should be elicited before dismissing a polypoidal defect in the cecum as an appendectomy defect.

References

General

Nahum H, Fékété F, Margulis AR: Radiology of the Postoperative Digestive Tract. New York, Masson Publishing, 1979.

Hiatus Hernia

Feigin DS, James AE Jr, Stitik FP, Donner MW, Skinner DB: The radiological appearance of hiatal hernia repairs. Radiology 110:71–77, 1974.
Skucas J, Mangea JC, Adams JT, Cutcliff W: An evaluation of the Nissen fundoplication. Radiology 118:539–544, 1976.
Teixidor HS, Evans JA: Roentgenographic appearance of the distal esophagus and the stomach after hiatal hernia repair. Am J Roentgenol 119:245–258, 1977.
Thoeni RF, Moss AA: The radiographic appearance of complications following Nissen fundoplication. Radiology 131:59–64, 1979.

Stomach Technique

Burhenne HJ: Roentgen anatomy and terminology of gastric surgery. Am J Roentgenol 91:731–743, 1964.
Burhenne HJ: Postoperative defects of the stomach. Semin Roentgenol 6:182–192, 1971.
Dunphy JE: Third Walter B. Cannon Lecture, 1974: The surgical treatment of gastrointestinal ulcer: past and future. Am J Roentgenol 123:229–235, 1975.

Gold RP, Seaman WB: The primary double-contrast examination of the postoperative stomach. Radiology 124:297–306, 1977.
Jay BS, Burrell M: Iatrogenic problems following gastric surgery. Gastrointest Radiol 2:239–257, 1977.
Ominsky SH, Moss AA: The postoperative stomach: a comparative study of double-contrast barium examinations and endoscopy. Gastrointest Radiol 4:17–22, 1979.
Op den Orth JO: Tubeless hypotonic examination of the afferent loop of the Billroth II stomach. Gastrointest Radiol 2:1–5, 1977.

Carcinoma in the Postoperative Stomach

Berk RN, Loeb PM, Miao YSF: Carcinoma of the gastric stump. J Can Assoc Radiol 25:127–130, 1974.
Burrell M, Touloukian JS, Curtis AM: Roentgen manifestations of carcinoma in the gastric remnant. Gastrointest Radiol 5:331–342, 1980.
Feldman F, Seaman WB: Primary gastric stump cancer. Am J Roentgenol 115:257–267, 1972.

Vagotomy

Bloch C, Wolf BS: The gastroduodenal channel after pyloroplasty and vagotomy: a cineradiographic study. Radiology 84:43–51, 1965.
Lewicki AM, Kleinhaus U, Brooks JR, Membreno AA: The small bowel following pyloroplasty and vagotomy. Radiology 109:539–544, 1973.

Jejunal Bypass

Moss AM, Goldbert GI, Koehler RE: Radiographic evaluation of complications after jejunoilial bypass surgery. Am J Roentgenol 127:737–741, 1976.

Appendectomy

Ekberg O: Cecal changes following appendectomy. Gastrointest Radiol 2:57–60, 1977.
Leadbetter GW Jr, Zickerman P, Pierce E: Ureterosigmoidostomy and carcinoma of the colon. J Urol 121:732–735, 1979.

11

PSEUDOLESIONS

The examination of the gastrointestinal tract may present many pitfalls in diagnosis for the beginner. There are many ways in which a lesion can be simulated when none is actually present. Until an internal standard of normality is developed, *everything* looks abnormal.

A number of basic principles are useful in helping to decide whether, for example, a projection is an artifact produced by peristalsis or a real lesion, or whether a narrowed area is indeed a lesion or is produced by spasm or some other artificial means.

Characteristics of Pseudolesions

The most important fact to keep in mind about pseudolesions is that they are *inconstant* (Fig. 11–1). Real lesions are always present;

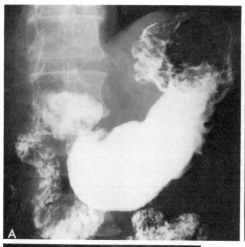 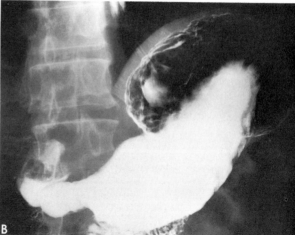

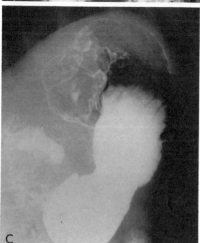

Figure 11–1. *A,* A filling defect in the fundus is created by the loose attachment of the mucosa and submucosa at the gastroesophageal junction. *B,* A subsequent film does not show any abnormality. *C,* Compare this film with multiple filling defects within the fundus due to gastric varices.

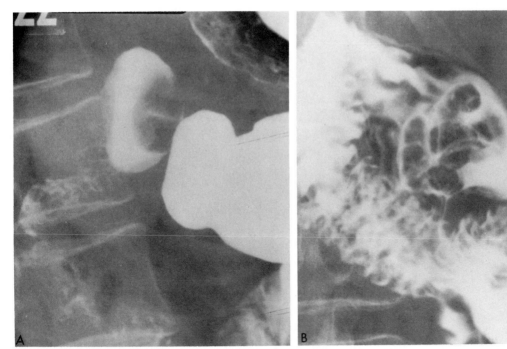

Figure 11–2. *A,* There is a smooth, *symmetrical* filling defect like a mushroom or umbrella at the base of the duodenal bulb; this represents prolapse of pyloric mucosa through the pyloric canal and is not indicative of disease. *B,* Multiple rounded, *asymmetrical* filling defects are seen in the base of the duodenal bulb, which represent actual sessile polyps. A filling defect at the base of the bulb may also be caused by a gastric polyp on a stalk prolapsing into the duodenum.

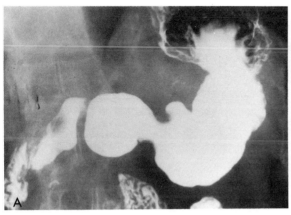

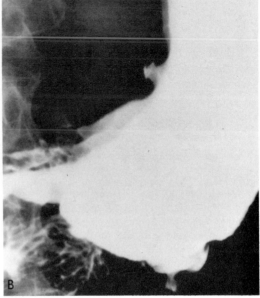

Figure 11–3. *A,* A large bulge is noted at the angularis, which is inconstant, changes in shape, and represents the membrana angularis defect in the gastric musculature. *B,* A constant projection is seen in this region. It has a surrounding halo and represents an ulcer crater.

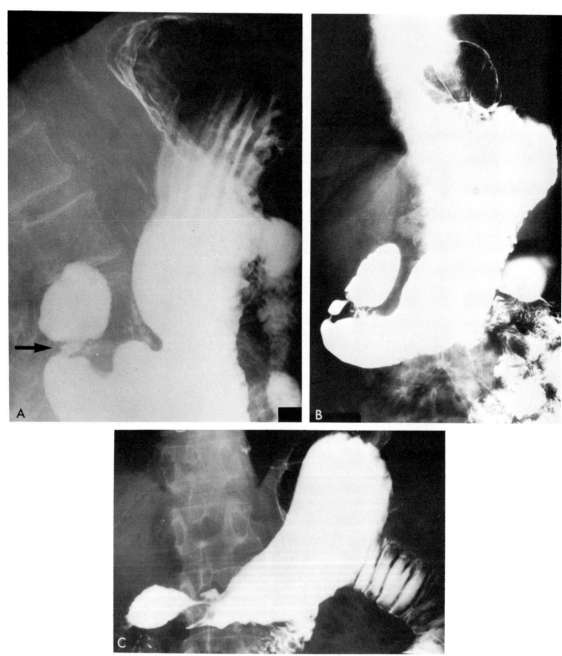

Figure 11–4. *A,* A bulge is seen on the greater curvature in the pyloric canal (arrow) — it is the "torus defect" due to the slinglike arrangement of the pyloric muscles. *B,* In hypertrophic pyloric stenosis, this torus defect is particularly well developed. One can see also that the pyloric canal is narrower than usual and is elongated beyond the normal length of 1 cm. Note also the large sliding hiatus hernia. *C,* A true pyloric canal ulcer is constant, will not change shape, and is squared off. Note the deformity of the greater curvature opposite the ulcer, with folds radiating to the ulcer crater. (Please note that these have been reproduced anatomically, although all are in fact prone films.)

they are seen on every film and can be reproduced with ease. A pseudolesion is inconstant, does not appear on every film, and cannot be reproduced easily.

NORMAL ENTITIES SIMULATING DISEASE

Fluid-Filled Fundus

One of the commonest pseudotumors within the abdomen is the fluid-filled fundus of the stomach. This is seen only when the patient is supine and should not be confused with a tumor of the left adrenal gland. Similarly, the duodenal bulb viewed end-on may mimic a mass in the right upper quadrant, and a fluid-filled loop of sigmoid colon may appear to be a mass in the pelvis.

Peristalsis

Peristalsis and the orientation of the underlying muscle may result in confusing constrictions or projections. Due to attenuation of all three muscle layers in the region of the angularis of the stomach, often a bulge appears between the angularis and the pylorus, which can be mistaken for an ulcer (Fig. 11–3). Similarly, at the pylorus, contraction of its slinglike muscles may cause a projection on either the greater or the lesser curvature, the so-called torus defect (Fig. 11–4). The clue that these are pseudoulcers and not real is, of course, the fact that these projections change in shape and are not seen on every film. If, however, they are persistent, a careful search should be made for concomitant peptic ulcer disease, as these bulges may become accentuated and more constant in the presence of acute inflammation. The torus defect becomes particularly prominent in conditions that cause hypertrophy of the pyloric muscle, e.g., adult hypertrophic pyloric stenosis.

Pyloric Canal

Another cause for confusion in the region of the pylorus is mistaking the pyloric canal

itself for an ulcer. The canal may be seen as either a collection of barium, a ring, or a star with radiating folds (Fig. 11–5). A similar appearance may be seen in the fundus of the stomach owing to the appearance of the gastroesophageal junction, the "rosette."

"Stricture" from Bending

When a tube bends, an apparent stricture or narrowing can be caused at the bend. This is a common cause of confusion in the small bowel, which, because of its length, has many curves and bends. Again, however, the clue to the fact that this is not organic disease is that the areas change in appearance. A specific pseudolesion due to kinking can be seen at the junction of the duodenal bulb and descending duodenum, the so-called "flexural pseudolesion" or pseudotumor. This is seen as a circular filling defect with a central collection of barium on the inner aspect of the duodenal flexure (Fig. 11–6); it is due to bunching of redundant duodenal mucosa. The "lesion" may be brought out by graded compression, and views in different obliquities will reveal that it is not a true lesion. This appearance can be simulated in other parts of the gut as well.

Colonic Strictures

In the colon, pseudostrictures occur at a number of specific sites. Some of these are due to localized thickening of the longitudinal and circular muscle fibers; others show no recognizable muscular thickening, and these areas of narrowing are presumably due to overactive neural impulses. It is, of course, important to differentiate these "strictured" areas from organic disease by showing that these do, indeed, relax (Fig. 11–7). An antispasmodic such as glucagon is extremely useful under these circumstances and should be used if a narrowed area is encountered anywhere in the GI tract. This will clarify whether the narrowing is actually caused by spasm or represents a real stricture. Similarly, nondistention from underfilling may create an appearance in the small bowel that simulates

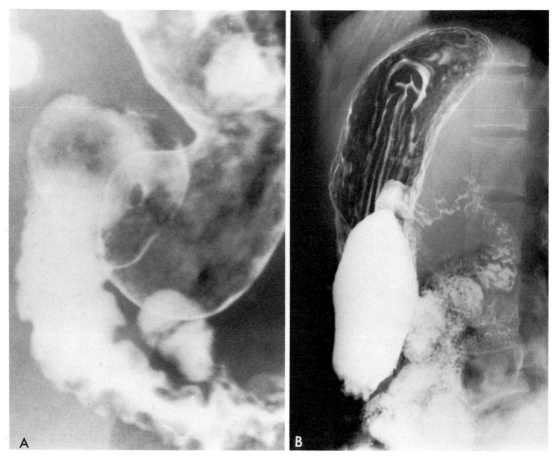

Figure 11–5. *A,* Any canal seen end-on can look like a round barium collection or a ring. If you see the mucosal folds extending to the canal, it will look like a star or radiating folds; misinterpreting these findings would result in false diagnosis of an ulcer. *B,* Note the rosette appearance of the gastroesophageal junction seen en face. The rosette is the commonest appearance of the cardia; variants include a circle and a hood. Distortion or enlargement of the rosette should suggest an abnormality.

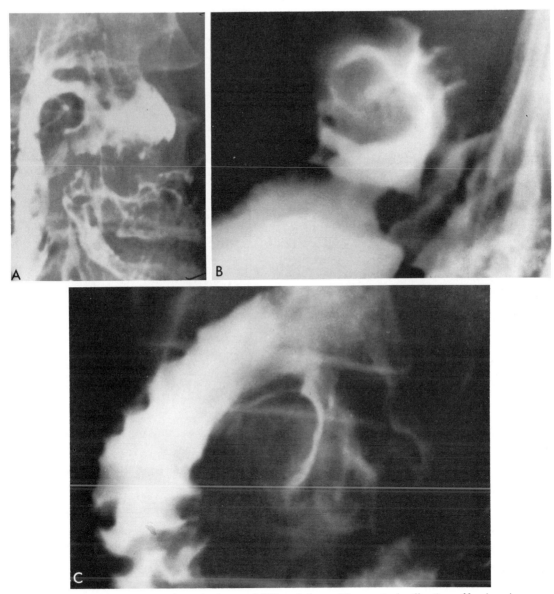

Figure 11–6. *Duodenal pseudoulcer. A,* A round filling defect with a central collection of barium is seen on the inner curve of the apex of the duodenal bulb. This represents stretching of mucosa over the underlying submucosa and crinkling of the associated folds. Do not mistake it for a real ulcer. *B,* If the pseudopolyp is seen "down the barrel," it will appear like a round filling defect. *C,* Unwinding the bulb and C-sweep shows that the "lesion" is not real, but instead is caused by the acute angle the C-sweep makes with the bulb. Note that in all three projections the duodenal bulb is not deformed, nor does it have any other evidence of inflammation.

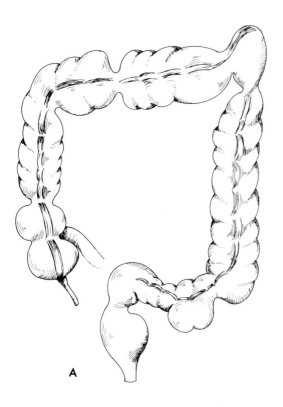

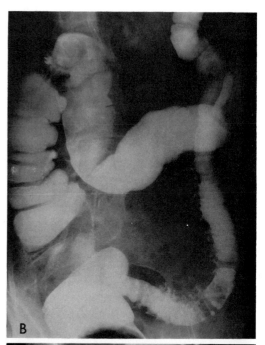

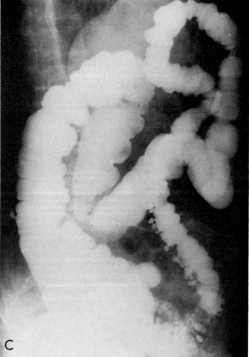

Figure 11–7. *A,* Multiple areas of narrowing are depicted — the so-called colonic sphincters. The radiologist must be aware of these and not confuse them with disease; it is, however, necessary to *prove* that these are not real applecore lesions, as is demonstrated by radiographs *B* and *C.*

B, A narrow area is seen at the hepatic flexure; an infiltrating lesion must be excluded by showing that it changes in caliber.

C, Following an intravenous injection of glucagon the "applecore" relaxes, revealing normal haustration and distention. This is the procedure to follow if a constricting "lesion" is suspected or if the narrowing is thought to be spasm and not disease.

ischemia. The underfilled leading edge of the barium column is also renowned for creating "disease" that disappears when that loop is fully distended. One must be careful not to diagnose an "applecore" lesion on a postevacuation film, for example, but to assess luminal diameter when the bowel is distended.

Background Pattern

It is important to recognize the normal background pattern of both the stomach and colon because to the uninitiated these may also simulate disease. The areae gastricae (Fig. 11–8) vary tremendously in appearance from patient to patient, but if they vary in size and shape in a single patient, gastritis should be suspected. The normal colon on air contrast is featureless; sometimes circular lines termed the innominate grooves (Fig. 11–9) are visible; these are seen especially when the colon is incompletely distended. In profile, these spiculations can simulate ulcerations. Circular rings can also occur in the esophagus, resulting in the "striped esophagus" recently reported in scleroderma.

Lymphoid Hyperplasia

Small, 1 to 2 mm nodular filling defects are commonly seen on double contrast enemas and should not be confused with disease; they represent lymphoid hyperplasia (Fig. 11–10). It is important to differentiate these from true nodules or polyps. In the duodenal bulb, not only can lymphoid hyperplasia be seen, but also other nonpathologic nodular defects, hypertrophied Brunner's glands, can be identified.

Foreign Bodies

Another confusing "lesion" can be caused by foreign bodies. This is most commonly the result of ingested food and, indeed, gastric polyps may be simulated by adherent food (Fig. 11–11). Undigested food such as bean sprouts (Fig. 11–12) or peas may be seen more distally and present equally confusing appearances. In the colon, of course, adherent feces must be differentiated from polyps (Fig. 11–12); to aid in this distinction the characteristic appearance of a sessile polyp has been

Text continued on page 183

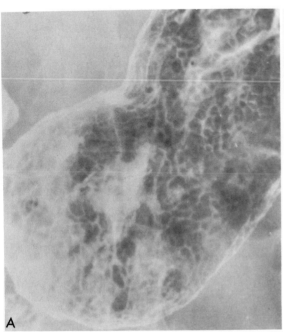

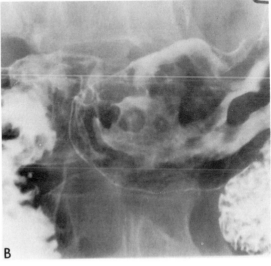

Figure 11–8. *A*, The fine lacelike pattern represents the normal surface pattern of the stomach, the areae gastricae; these should not be confused with a network of erosions, which would be collections of barium with a surrounding rim due to the edema mound, as is seen in *B*.

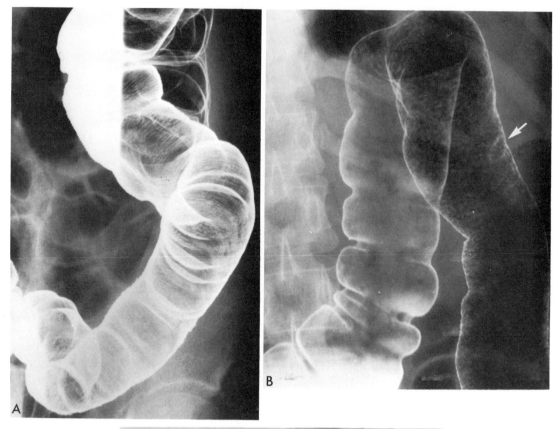

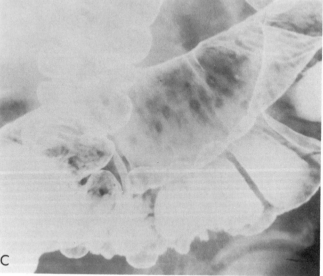

Figure 11–9. *A,* The circular lines in the descending colon and sigmoid are the normal background pattern of the colon, the innominate grooves. These spiculations along the edge of the air column should not be confused with mucosal ulcers.

B, Contrast this appearance with that in *B* and *C.* In *B,* there is a granular background pattern due to ulcerative colitis, with fine spiculation to the edge of the barium; the colon proximal to the splenic flexure is normal. A postinflammatory polyp is seen distal to the splenic flexure (arrow).

C, Multiple discrete aphthoid ulcers are present in the sigmoid colon. These superficial ulcers, which have a surrounding halo of edema, are characteristic of Crohn's disease.

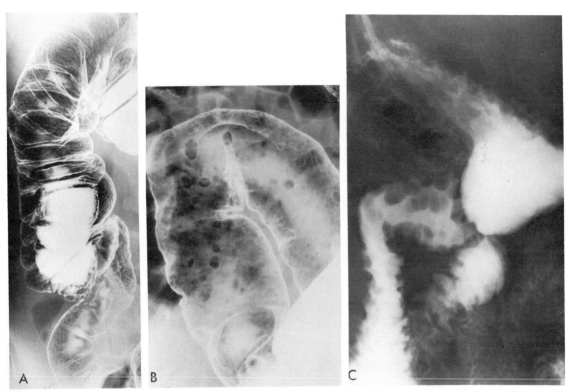

Figure 11–10. *A*, Tiny, round filling defects in the right colon and terminal ileum represent lymphoid hyperplasia. These are uniform in size (1 to 2 mm in diameter) and form a sheet. This appearance should not be confused with that of multiple polyps *(B)*, which vary in size and shape. *C*, Multiple filling defects in the duodenal bulb can represent either lymphoid hyperplasia or, more commonly, Brunner gland hyperplasia, as is shown here, the nodular defects being about 1 cm in size.

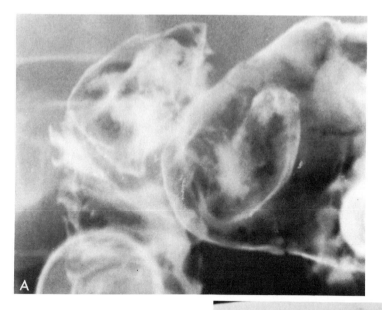

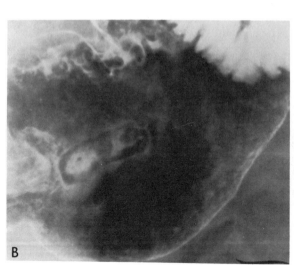

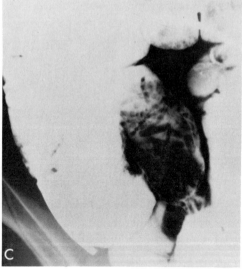

Figure 11–11. *A,* Adherent food can be misdiagnosed as an intraluminal tumor. In a diabetic patient with gastric atrophy, a filling defect in the antrum was diagnosed as a tumor; no lesion was found at endoscopy and a follow-up study after prolonged fasting and gastric aspiration showed completely normal results.

B, A rectangular filling defect is seen in the stomach as a result of a nondigested bean. The nonanatomic nature of the filling defect is the clue that this is not a real lesion.

C, Multiple *linear* filling defects are present in the terminal ileum. The patient had eaten a meal of Chinese food the night before the examination; these filling defects represent undigested bean sprouts. The shape should suggest that these are artifacts and not polyps, although you must keep in mind the unusually shaped filiform polyp of inflammatory bowel disease (see Figure 11–13D). (By courtesy of Francis J. Scholz, Lahey Clinic, Boston.)

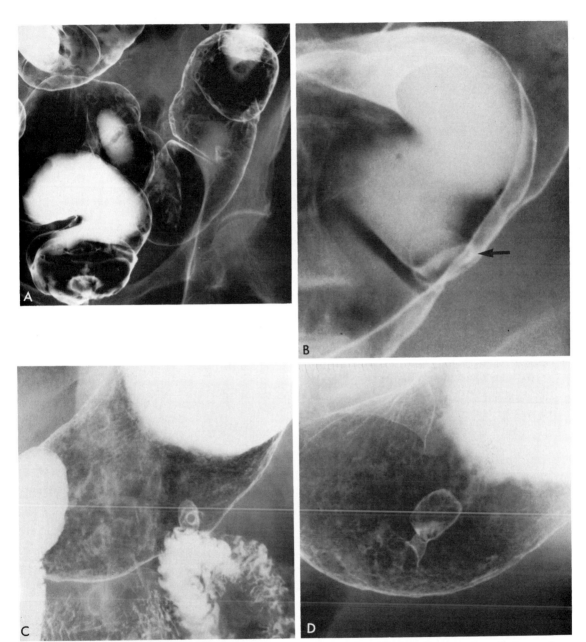

Figure 11–12. *A,* Adherent feces in the colon (or foreign bodies) can be a real source of confusion and can be difficult to differentiate from real lesions. Sometimes the irregular shape of the filling defects indicates stool and not round polyps. *B,* The "bowler hat" sign (arrow) is said to represent a real lesion and not to be seen with stool. *C,* Similarly, the "Mexican hat" sign represents a real lesion and results from looking directly down on a polyp along its stalk. The smaller circle within the larger circle is the stalk seen on-end. *D,* The stalk is easily demonstrated by turning the patient oblique.

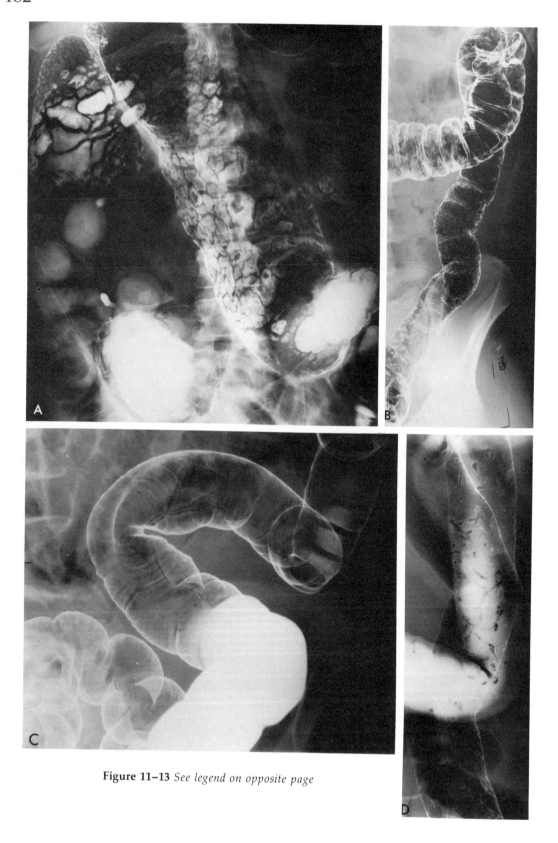

Figure 11–13 *See legend on opposite page*

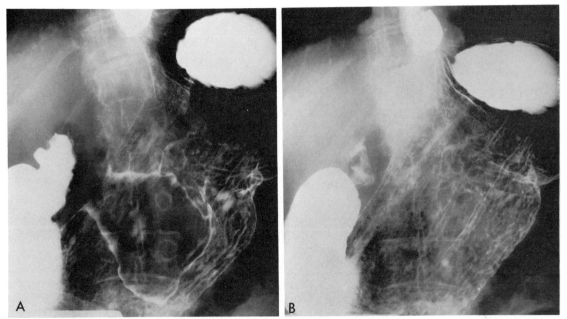

Figure 11–14. *A*, "Lesions" may be created by lack of distention during air contrast work when the two opposite walls stick together, the so-called "kissing walls." Compression on the stomach will produce these artifacts and they will be abolished by releasing the compression or by obtaining more distention, as in *B*. Note the distorted fold pattern just above the kissing wall defect, which is due to a shallow ulcer on the anterior wall of the stomach.

described, termed the "bowler hat" sign. Gas bubbles and mucus strands may also cause problems and should not be confused with real lesions (Fig. 11–13).

"Kissing Walls"

The air contrast technique itself may result in a number of traps. In this method added lines or crescents are sought in the air-distended, barium-coated viscus. The two opposing walls may stick together, resulting in false lines, the so-called "kissing walls" (Fig. 11–14). This may be produced transiently by using compression and will disappear when compression is released. If this is suspected, it can be abolished by obtaining more distention.

Hanging Droplet

The hanging droplet or stalactite phenomenon may be responsible for a false diagnosis of ulcerated polyps (target lesions) (Fig. 11–

Figure 11–13. *A*, "Lesions" can be created by the effect of intraluminal contents on the barium. Excess mucus can result in a "crocodile skin" appearance, or even an appearance that can simulate mucosal ulcers.

B, Note how the mottled effect in the descending colon due to barium flocculation could be misdiagnosed as the coarse granularity of ulcerative colitis.

C, Characteristic mucus strands are seen in the sigmoid and descending colon; occasionally long strands of mucus can be mistaken for the stalk of a polyp.

D, Not all linear filling defects can be dismissed as mucus. Filiform polyps are real lesions, are rectangular in shape, and follow bad attacks of either ulcerative colitis or Crohn's disease; they must be differentiated from the mucus strands in *C*.

15). A common mistake is to confuse a collection of barium in the center of a nondependent polyp with an ulcer.

"Shine-Through" Artifacts

It may sound simplistic, but "shine-through" artifacts can be a problem, especially with the air contrast technique; a rib or the sacroiliac joint viewed obliquely may simulate the stalk of a polyp, and it is very embarrassing if one mistakes a vertebral pedicle for a polyp (Fig. 11–16). The enema tip itself has round holes in it, which should not be con-

fused with polyps. Pseudolesions can be created by the enema tip balloon, and repeat films of the rectum should always be done after the balloon has been deflated.

Postoperative Defects

Postoperative defects or pseudotumors may present another problem. All radiologists are familiar with the problem of differentiating between postpyloroplasty bulges and active duodenal ulcers, but occasionally actual tumors may be mimicked by surgery. One of the commonest is the "tumor" created in the

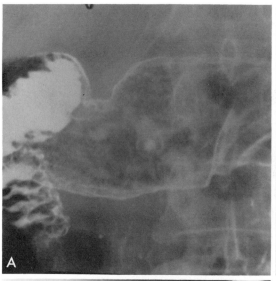

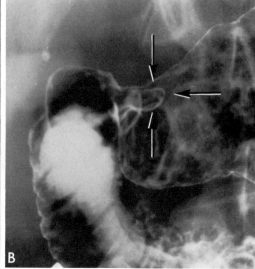

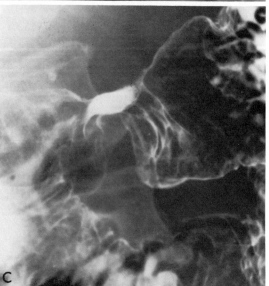

Figure 11–15. *A,* A "target" lesion is seen in the antrum, which might result in a false diagnosis of an ulcerated polyp. Analyze, however, on which wall it is — the nondependent surface (if it were dependent it would be a filling defect in a pool of barium). The central "ulcer" is a pseudolesion and due to the "hanging droplet" or stalactite phenomenon. Compare this appearance with *B;* this shows the "empty ulcer" sign observed when the ulcer has emptied of its pool of barium leaving a ring (arrows). This can be proved to be an ulcer if it fills with barium on turning the patient (as in *C). (B* and *C* by courtesy of Francis J. Scholz, Lahey Clinic, Boston.)

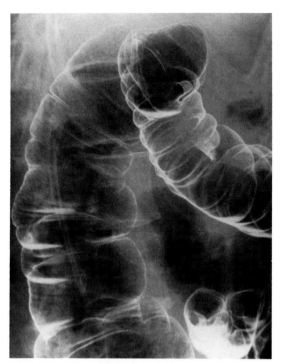

Figure 11–16. Normal structures projected through the distended organ can be mistaken for lesions. The oblique white lines represent not the stalk of a polyp but a rib projected over the air column. Similarly, the sacroiliac joints can mimic a stalk and a pedicle or sacral foramen may look like a sessile polyp. Incidentally, note the extrinsic defect on the hepatic flexure caused by the gallbladder.

gastric fundus by a Nissen fundoplication when the gastric fundus is wrapped around the distal esophagus as an antireflux procedure. This may be seen on a plain film and should not be confused with, say, a leiomyoma of the fundus. Similarly, the inturned appendiceal stump should not be confused with a cecal polyp; characteristically, the defect is inferior to the ileocecal valve and on the medial wall (see Chapter 10).

Postoperative Inflammation

If tubes or drains have been left in place, a localized bulge or tethered area may simulate inflammation or ulceration; this is quite common following gastrostomy.

In summary, each radiologist must build up in his or her own mind a mental image of the range of normality. After a while the eye will immediately dismiss most of these pseudolesions. Others will take a little analyzing, but that's half the fun; otherwise life would be too easy.

References

Bremner CG: The lesser curve pyloric niche. Br J Radiol 41:291–295, 1968.

Burrell M, Toffler R: Flexural pseudolesions of the duodenum. Radiology 120:313–315, 1976.

Calenoff L, Sparberg M: Gastric pseudolesions: roentgenographic-gastrophotographic correlation. Am J Roentgenol 113:139–146, 1971.

Cole FM: Innominate grooves of the colon: morphological characteristics and etiologic mechanisms. Radiology 128:41–43, 1978.

de Lorimier AA, Warren JP: Prolapse of the mucosa at the esophagogastric junction. Am J Roentgenol 84:1061–1069, 1960.

Ekberg O: Cecal changes following appendectomy. Gastrointest Radiol 2:57–60, 1977.

Feigin DS, James AE Jr, Stitik FP, Donner MW, Skinner DB: The radiological appearance of hiatal hernia repairs. Radiology 110:71–77, 1974.

Franken EA Jr: Lymphoid hyperplasia of the colon. Radiology 94:329–334, 1970.

Freeny PC: Double-contrast gastrography of the fundus and cardia: normal landmarks and their pathologic changes. Am J Roentgenol 133:481–488, 1979.

Gohel VK, Kressel HY, Laufer I: Double-current artifacts. Gastrointest Radiol 3:139–146, 1978.

Kelvin FM, Max RJ, Norton GA, Oddson TA, Rice RP, Thompson WM, Garbutt JT: Lymphoid follicular pattern of the colon in adults. Am J Roentgenol 133:821–826, 1979.

Langkemper R, Hoek AC, Dekker W, Op den Orth JO: Elevated lesions in the duodenal bulb caused by heterotopic gastric mucosa. Radiology 137:621–624, 1980.

Matsuura K, Nakata H, Takeda N, Nakata S, Shimoda Y: Innominate lines of the colon. Radiology 123:581–584, 1977.

Nelson JA, Sheft DJ, Minagi H, Ferruci JT Jr: Duodenal pseudopolyp — the flexure fallacy. Am J Roentgenol 123:262–267, 1975.

Op den Orth JO, Ploem S: The stalactite phenomenon in double contrast studies of the stomach. Radiology 117:523–525, 1975.

Peavy PW, Clements JL Jr, Weens HS: Gastric pseudo-ulcers: membrana angularis and pyloric torus defects. Radiology 114:591–595, 1975.

Skucas J, Mangla JC, Adams JJ, Cutliff W: An evaluation of the Nissen fundoplication. Radiology 118:539–544, 1976.

Templeton AW: Colon sphincters simulating organic disease. Radiology 75:237–241, 1960.

Williams I: Innominate grooves in the surface of mucosa. Radiology 84:877–880, 1965.

Youker JE, Welin S: Differentiation of true polypoid tumors of the colon from extraneous material: a new roentgen sign. Radiology 84:610–615, 1965.

12

COMMON IATROGENIC COMPLICATIONS

Iatrogenic complications are being seen more frequently with today's aggressive diagnostic and therapeutic interventions. This is as true for the gastrointestinal tract as it is for other systems. Iatrogenic causes probably should be thought of more frequently than they are, and if the right questions are asked and an adequate history obtained, the radiologist may be able to identify a potentially reversible complication.

DRUGS

Many classes of drugs adversely affect the gastrointestinal tract; some complications present fairly characteristic x-ray appearances. Drug effects can be considered under several broad categories: drugs that affect motility, those that induce inflammation or fibrosis, those that induce bleeding or thrombosis, and those that cause an alteration in the normal

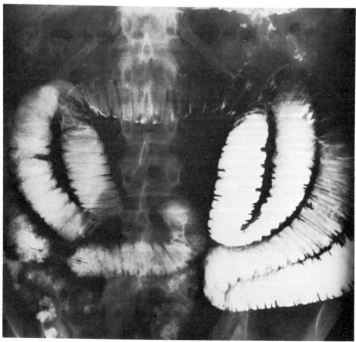

Figure 12–1. *Small bowel stricture due to enteric-coated potassium preparations (slow-K).* The small bowel is dilated because of partial obstruction; there is a stricture (arrows) in the mid to distal small bowel. At surgery this was found to be a benign stricture; the patient had been taking diuretics and slow-K supplements.

bowel flora. Some of the classic appearances in each of these categories will be illustrated.

Many drugs are known to be ulcerogenic, including aspirin, steroids, and other anti-inflammatory agents. A severe complication used to be associated with enteric-coated potassium chloride (Fig. 12–1); ulcers and strictures involving the small bowel were brought about by slow release and prolonged contact with this potent chemical. Banning the offending preparations has prevented many of these complications.

Bowel motility can be affected by many drugs. Narcotics and other, similar pain relievers decrease motility and produce ileus. Psychoactive drugs can potentiate a particularly severe form of atony, pseudo-obstruction. The radiographic appearance can be quite alarming, and further diagnostic workup or even surgery may be necessary to exclude a mechanical obstruction. An accurate drug history can enable the radiologist to include this in the differential diagnosis.

Anticoagulants are potent medications requiring careful titration of dosage, and there are many examples of intramural hemorrhage secondary to anticoagulant mismanagement. The appearance of an intramural bleed is characteristic; knowing the appropriate drug history is helpful for prompt diagnosis and treatment. Even if the medication is carefully controlled, unsuspected lesions (for example, an asymptomatic ulcer) may present with acute bleeding when the patient is put on anticoagulant therapy (Fig. 12–2). The radiologist is often asked to exclude an active ulcer in the patient with a history of ulcer disease before the patient is started on anticoagulation. Similarly, the radiologist is often asked to find the source when the patient on anticoagulation suddenly begins to bleed.

Several well-known, widely used drugs can cause ischemia of the bowel. Contraceptives are known to cause ischemia, which is usually reversible. The widespread use of these agents should alert the radiologist to possible complications. Another extremely important drug has also been associated with ischemic changes of bowel: digitalis. This drug induces nonobstructive ischemia, the so-called low-flow state. This complication is

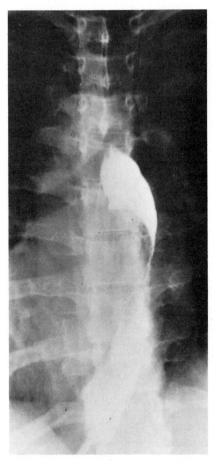

Figure 12–2. *Intramural hematoma.* A large intramural (note the relatively acute angle of take-off) filling defect is present in a patient on Coumadin therapy. The lesion resolved spontaneously.

most often seen in elderly patients who already have circulatory compromise.

Cathartics, widely used and frequently abused, are responsible for chronic colonic changes. "Cathartic colon" (Fig. 12–3) has a remarkable x-ray appearance, which can be confused on quick glance with chronic ulcerative colitis if certain features, such as colon length, are not taken into account.

Prolonged use of methysergide (Sansert) can cause retroperitoneal fibrosis, which most often affects the ureters, resulting in obstruction. GI tract manifestations are rare, but there are occasional reports of extrinsic compression of bowel in the pelvis or ischemia secondary to mesenteric vascular compression.

More aggressive chemotherapy for many malignancies has brought with it an increase

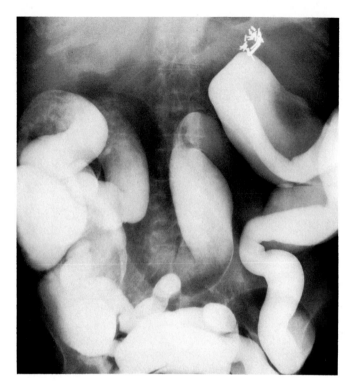

Figure 12–3. *"Cathartic colon."* The colon is ahaustral but very redundant, a characteristic appearance suggesting cathartic abuse. This should not be confused with chronic inflammatory disease, in which the ahaustral colon is also shortened.

in opportunistic infections, many of which manifest themselves in the lungs. Perhaps the most dramatic GI manifestation associated with immunosuppression is esophageal candidiasis. *Candida albicans* is part of the normal flora, but the marked overgrowth sometimes seen in immunosuppressed patients has a characteristic x-ray appearance. The esophagus is irritable and spastic, the mucosa shaggy and ulcerated, and the ulcers are frequently linear; filling defects due to the monilial plaques (Fig. 12–4) may be seen. Note should be made that with mild disease the study may be normal, so candidiasis is not necessarily excluded by a normal examination. This is particularly true if a single contrast examination is performed; a double contrast examination of the esophagus is helpful in diagnosing early, subtle changes.

Antibiotics are usually thought of as medications of unparalleled value, but their toxicity is also well appreciated. Perhaps the most virulent GI manifestation is pseudomembranous colitis. Patients taking certain antibiotics (among them clindamycin) suddenly manifest diarrhea and fever. Sigmoidoscopy and barium enema are diagnostic. Ulcerated, friable mucosa covered by a shaggy pseudomembrane is diagnostic. Submucosal edema/

hemorrhage is a component feature, as are plaque-like lesions.

One curious therapeutic complication has been reported. Proteolytic enzymes such as papain have been used to dissolve a meat bolus that has impacted in the distal esophagus. This drug has been known to dissolve not only the meat, but also the esophagus, resulting in perforation.

Even this brief introduction should serve to remind the radiologist of the wide range of drug toxicity and how frequently there are radiographic manifestations. One point should be stressed again: to diagnose iatrogenic disease the radiologist must keep its possibility in mind.

RADIATION

Radiation can damage normal as well as abnormal tissue (Fig. 12–5). Radiotherapists must tread a narrow path between benefit and toxicity. Because of rapid cell turnover, most of the gastrointestinal tract is relatively radiosensitive. The esophagus is particularly vulnerable, not only because it is very radiosensitive, but also because it is included in mediastinal treatment fields for commonly irradiated thoracic malignancies. Disordered motility is seen early, and smooth, benign-appearing strictures can be a late feature. The stomach is less frequently involved, but pre-pyloric ulcers and deformities are known complications. The small bowel, although frequently irradiated, is protected to some extent by its mobility. However, complications, frequently life-threatening, may arise if bowel is irradiated while it is trapped in one place, as for instance by adhesion or inflammation, commonly in the pelvis. As a consequence the wide spectrum of radiation enteritis can be produced. Radiation can be thought of as an inflammatory process that induces edema. Common manifestations of radiation enteritis include thickened folds, luminal narrowing and fixation, matting, and angulation of loops; obstruction and fistulae may occur. Radiation injury to the colon is manifested typically by a smooth, elongated stricture. When the colonic anatomy (as defined by pretreatment barium enema) is known, proper treatment planning can minimize this complication.

Endoscopy

Endoscopy of the GI tract has become an important diagnostic tool with its own well-documented complications, the most dangerous of which is perforation. Esophageal perforations can occur high in the cervical area or distally; in either case, potentially fatal infection can supervene. Pneumatic dilatation of an esophageal stricture can also result in perforation. Perforation of the stomach can occur most easily through the posterior wall, and large volumes of air and fluid will then enter the lesser sac. Perforation of any organ is more likely if the endoscope is passing through diseased gut or if a biopsy is also performed. The new flexible endoscopes have been known to retroflex inadvertently and become impacted when an attempt is made to remove them. One alarming complication of endoscopy has been reported: the pseudo–acute abdomen. This is caused by a large volume of insufflated air which, particularly in small bowel, results in severe abdominal cramping and distention. The first assumption is that a viscus has perforated. An abdominal series will show the intraluminal location of massive amounts of air, obviating surgical intervention.

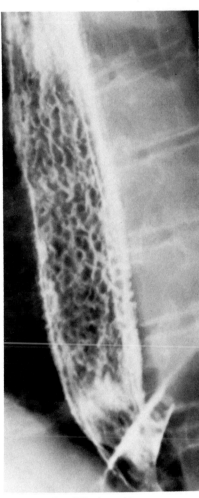

Figure 12–4. *Candidiasis.* Air contrast barium swallow shows multiple projections with collections of barium consistent with ulcers. In addition, there are multiple filling defects due to the fungal plaques. Sometimes the patient is in too much pain to be able to swallow the heavy barium preparation and gas needed for an air contrast examination. Spasm and irritability may be the only abnormal findings. (Courtesy of Francis J. Scholz, Lahey Clinic, Boston, MA.)

Tubes

A myriad of tubes can be introduced into the patient, frequently with dire consequences. Perforation of the esophagus is not unheard of, even with a soft nasogastric tube, especially in the infant. Nasogastric tubes

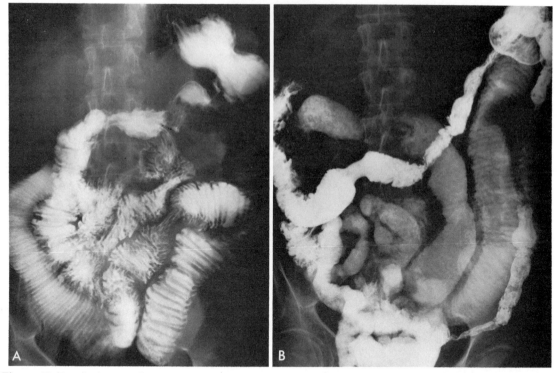

Figure 12–5. *A, Acute radiation enteritis.* Small bowel follow-through shows some thickening of the folds in a picket-fence configuration in the right lower quadrant. This appearance is due to submucosal inflammation and edema.

B, Chronic radiation change. A small bowel follow-through some 6 months later shows that the affected area is more extensive than previously thought. The affected loops now appear featureless and dilated. There is some evidence of malabsorption (dilution).

have been reported to result in esophageal stricture, perhaps secondary to the reflux they induce. Traumatic passage of a tube can cause a submucosal hemorrhage, which can compromise the lumen. Obviously, trauma, including perforation, is more easily induced with large bore tubes, such as the Sengstaken-Blakemore tube used to tamponade bleeding esophageal varices; improper positioning of the balloons can contribute to complications.

Tubes can knot in the lumen of the gut and can cause trouble at removal time. Plain films or fluoroscopy frequently can reveal the problem. Long tubes equipped with mercury bags are more prone to knotting because of their redundancy. In addition, it is possible for the bag to leak or perforate, spilling mercury into the gut. Although this produces an alarming x-ray appearance, it is apparently a benign complication.

SURGERY

Alimentary tract surgery is so diverse that it is impossible to catalogue all potential complications here. Most of the surgical material has been dealt with in the chapter on postoperative radiology, but a brief review is in order. It should be remembered that radiographically one can make the diagnosis of opaque foreign bodies, including instruments and sponges; sponges used in the operating room contain a radiopaque strip that make them easily visible. As already mentioned, surgical complications include anastomotic leaks early in the postoperative period and stricture formation later in life. This is true whether the operation is performed on the esophagus, stomach, small bowel, or colon. Poor drainage from the stomach following gastric resection can set the stage for bezoar formation; large conglomerations of hair or cellulose can coalesce into a large foreign body, causing both satiety and obstructive symptoms.

Perhaps the most common iatrogenic problem related to the small bowel is obstruction secondary to adhesions. Another interesting problem is pneumatosis intestinalis following small bowel bypass for morbid obesity. A more lethal complication is aortoenteric fistula, which results when an infected graft erodes into small bowel or duodenum, causing massive gastrointestinal hemorrhage.

MISCELLANEOUS

Radiologists, too, have become more aggressive in both diagnosis and treatment; some complications of procedures have been the inevitable result. Balloon-tipped barium enema tubes are an example. This advancement in equipment has facilitated many a barium enema, especially in the older patient with poor rectal tone. Occasionally, however, overdistention of the balloon has resulted in laceration or perforation of the rectum (Fig. 12–6). The tube can be inadvertently inserted into the vagina. A potentially fatal adjunct to this perforation is venous intravasation of barium into pelvic veins, with subsequent barium embolization.

Water-soluble contrast media such as Gastrografin can induce pulmonary edema if aspirated into the lungs. Extreme care must be exercised in using this substance in moribund individuals.

It should be obvious that complications are inherent in many of the complex diagnostic and therapeutic interventions of modern medicine. The radiologist is ideally situated to recognize, evaluate, and perhaps even to help alleviate many of the iatrogenic problems discussed.

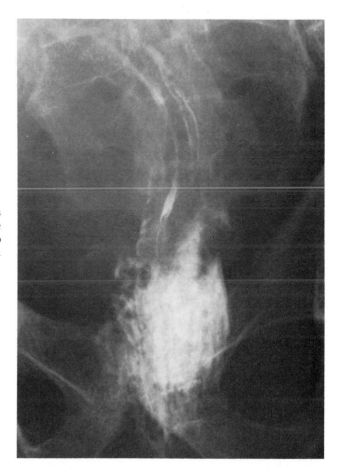

Figure 12–6. *Perforation of the rectum.* This postevacuation, coned-down view of the rectum shows an unusual configuration to the barium column; this represents barium within the muscle layers of the rectal wall.

References

General

Athey PA, Goldstein HM, Dodd GD: Radiologic spectrum of opportunistic infections of the upper gastrointestinal tract. Am J Roentgenol 129:419–424, 1977.

Gelfand DW: Complications of gastrointestinal radiologic procedures: I. Complications of routine fluoroscopic studies. Gastrointest Radiol 5:293, 1980.

Ghahremani GG, Turner MA, Port RB: Iatrogenic intubation injuries of the upper gastrointestinal tract in adults. Gastrointest Radiol 5:1, 1980.

Haskin M, Pais MJ, Haskin PH: Complications of routine gastrointestinal x-ray examination. Clearfield HR, Dinoso VP Jr: Gastrointestinal Emergencies. New York, Grune & Stratton, 1976, pp. 281–289.

Hunt TH, Gelfand DW: Complications of gastrointestinal radiologic procedures. III. Complications of diagnostic and interventional angiography. Gastrointest Radiol 6:57, 1981.

Hyson EA, Burrell M, Toffler R: Drug-induced gastrointestinal disease. Gastrointest Radiol 2:183–212, 1977.

Mettler FA Jr: Manifestations of drug toxicity. In Moseley RD Jr, Current Problems in Diagnostic Radiology. Vol. 13: Chicago, Year Book Medical Publishers, 1979.

Ott DJ, Gelfand DW: Complications of gastrointestinal radiologic procedures. II. Complications related to biliary tract studies. Gastrointest Radiol 6:47, 1981.

Rogers LF, Goldstein HM: Roentgen manifestations of radiation injury to the gastrointestinal tract. Gastrointest Radiol 2:281–291, 1977.

Roswit B: Complications of radiation therapy: the alimentary tract. Semin Roentgenol 9:51–63, 1974.

Esophagus

Calenoff L, Rogers LF: Radiologic manifestations of iatrogenic changes of the esophagus. Gastrointest Radiol 2:229–237, 1977.

Lewicki AM, Moore JP: Esophageal moniliasis. A review of common and less frequent characteristics. Am J Roentgenol 125:218, 1975.

Meyers C, Durkin MG, Love L: Radiographic findings in herpetic esophagitis. Radiology 119:21, 1976.

Meyers MA, Ghahremani GG: Complications of fiberoptic endoscopy. I. Esophagoscopy and gastroscopy. Radiology 115:293, 1975.

Small Bowel

Ghahremani GG, Meyers MA, Farman J, Port RB: Ischemic disease of the small bowel and colon associated with oral contraceptives. Gastrointest Radiol 2:221–228, 1977.

Thompson WM, Jackson DC, Johnsrude IS: Aortoenteric and para-prosthetic-enteric fistulas: radiologic findings. Am J Roentgenol 127:235–242, 1976.

Colon

Dodds WJ, Stewart ET, Nelson JA: Rectal balloon catheters and the barium enema examination. Gastrointest Radiol 5:277–284, 1980.

Meyers MA, Ghahremani GG: Complications of fiberoptic endoscopy. II. Colonscopy. Radiology 115:301, 1975.

Nelson JA, Daniels AU, Dodds WJ: Rectal balloons: complications, causes, and recommendations. Invest Radiol 14:48–59, 1979.

Pyle R, Samuel E: An evaluation of the hazards of barium enema examination. Clin Radiol 11:192–199, 1960.

Seaman WB, Wells J: Complications of the barium enema. Gastroenterology 48:728–737, 1965.

Stanley RJ, Melson GL, Tedesco FJ: The spectrum of radiographic findings in antibiotic-related pseudomembranous colitis. Radiology 111:519–524, 1974.

Stanley RJ, Melson GL, Tedesco FJ, Saylor JL: Plain-film findings in severe pseudomembranous colitis. Radiology 118:7, 1976.

Urso FP, Urso MJ, Lee CH: The cathartic colon: pathological findings and radiological/pathological correlation. Radiology 116:557, 1975.

13

THE BILIARY SYSTEM AND PANCREAS

A few years ago evaluating the biliary tree radiographically was a relatively simple matter; only a few techniques were available, and the choice was limited. Evaluation of the gallbladder was done by the oral cholecystogram (OCG) and of the hepatic and common ducts by the intravenous cholangiogram (IVC). If the patient was jaundiced, and the problem was to differentiate between "medical" and "surgical" jaundice, percutaneous transhepatic cholangiogram or endoscopic retrograde cholangiopancreatography (ERCP) (the so-called direct nonoperative cholangiographic techniques) was called into play. Nuclear medicine studies played a relatively minor role in defining the biliary tree, although ^{131}I rose bengal was used to try to differentiate patent from obstructed ducts.

In no site in gastrointestinal radiography have the newer cross-sectional techniques (ultrasound and computed tomography) and the newer radionuclide agents had a wider impact than in the evaluation of the biliary system. The simple choice of "what to do when" has therefore become blurred by the profusion of tests now available. Based on the principle of moving from noninvasive to invasive procedures when the noninvasive give equivocal results, approaches to various clinical situations will be suggested. A brief discussion of the pros and cons and do's and don't's in biliary disease is presented. Since pancreatic disease is usually discussed in conjunction with obstructive jaundice, an attempt will be made to follow this convention in a logical manner.

A number of pertinent questions may be asked in each clinical situation that will help in deciding how to proceed.

1. Is disease of the *gallbladder itself* or disease involving the *ducts* suspected?

2. Is the most likely diagnosis gallstones or pancreatic disease?

3. Is the patient *jaundiced* or not?

4. If the patient *is jaundiced,* is this due to liver disease (the so-called "medical" jaundice) or is it due to duct obstruction ("surgical" jaundice)? The aim of all tests in the jaundiced patient is to find out if the ducts are normal in size (presumed medical) or dilated (a presumably obstructed system).

5. Is the patient *acutely ill* with a suspected underlying inflammatory process, such as acute cholecystitis or cholangitis, or is this a process of *insidious onset*?

The available tests will now be discussed briefly, including how to judge which tests may be most helpful in various clinical situations.

PLAIN FILM OF THE ABDOMEN (KUB)

This may not be helpful in biliary disease, since relatively few gallstones (15 per cent)

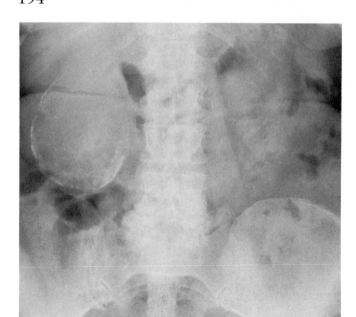

Figure 13–1. *Porcelain gallbladder.* The rim of calcification in the right upper quadrant represents a porcelain gallbladder; here the calcium is actually within the wall and this is a form of chronic cholecystitis. There is an increased risk of carcinoma of the gallbladder in this condition.

contain enough calcium to be visible on a plain film (Fig. 13–2). Occasionally a soft tissue mass in the right upper quadrant or pancreatic area, or pancreatic calcification, may be seen; gas may be present in the biliary tree.

ULTRASOUND AND COMPUTED TOMOGRAPHY

Ultrasound has become extremely popular as a screening procedure. In expert hands, the diagnosis of cholelithiasis (Fig. 13–3) can

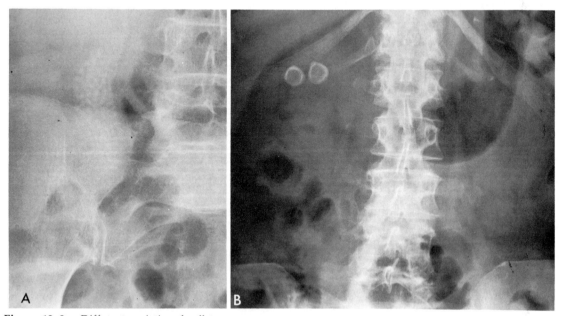

Figure 13–2. *Different varieties of gallstones.*
  A, Multiple tiny opacities are seen in the right upper quadrant. (The patient has not been given contrast medium.)
  B, *Lamellar gallstones.* Two concentric calcifications are seen in the right upper quadrant.

be 98 per cent accurate. It may also be helpful in the diagnosis of acute cholecystitis, particularly if (in addition to gallstones, especially one impacted in the cystic duct) one can demonstrate *probe tenderness* exactly over the gallbladder (sonographic Murphy's sign) or a thickened gallbladder wall. It is also highly accurate in assessing duct size (the normal size of the ducts on ultrasound is less than with contrast medium; common bile duct is 4 to 5 mm, intrahepatic ducts 3 to 4 mm). Its versatility lies in the fact that frequently the *etiology* of duct dilatation can be demonstrated at the same examination; for example, a mass in the head of the pancreas. However, differentiation between localized pancreatitis and carcinoma has been less successful than hoped for, and the technique is severely limited in many examinations by presence of intestinal gas.

The second cross-sectional imaging procedure, computed tomography, clearly and rapidly defines intra-abdominal structures, including the pancreas and biliary tree. It is, however, relatively expensive, and the radiation dose for multiple cuts is not inconsiderable. Its use should be reserved for those cases in which ultrasound is equivocal or unsuccessful. It is probably the preferred method for the evaluation of the retroperitoneum.

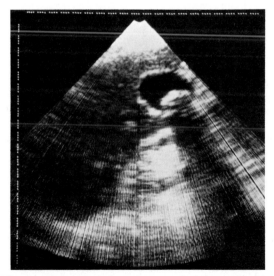

Figure 13–3. *Real-time ultrasound of the gallbladder* demonstrates a large calculus casting a prominent acoustic shadow.

TABLE 13–1. CAUSES OF NONVISUALIZATION OF THE GALLBLADDER

1. Vomiting, diarrhea or failure to take tablets
2. Retention of contrast medium within either esophagus (e.g., stricture) or stomach; if the sick patient is lying on his back, contrast medium will be retained in fundus of stomach
3. Malabsorption, e.g., that due to underlying disease, such as sprue, or following pancreatitis (it is recommended that an OCG be delayed 6 weeks following either acute cholecystitis or pancreatitis)
4. Liver disease
5. Gallbladder disease
   a. Acute cholecystitis (cystic duct obstruction)
   b. Acalculous cholecystitis
   c. Chronic cholecystitis
   d. Cholelithiasis

CONTRAST STUDIES OF THE BILIARY TREE

The oral cholecystogram is an extremely popular study, and some 40 million studies have been performed in the United States in the last 20 years. It is quoted as being 96 per cent accurate, and stones as small as 1 to 2 mm have been diagnosed, but at this tiny size many calculi must be missed. The oral cholecystogram is limited by liver function and one cannot expect visualization when the bilirubin level is above 2 per cent (2 mg/dl). It is not helpful in acute situations because the examination can take up to 48 hours to complete.

Opacification of the gallbladder depends upon a complex series of events, failure of any one of which will result in "nonvisualization" of the gallbladder (Table 13–1); this in effect is a false-positive diagnosis of gallbladder disease. The contrast medium must be (a) *absorbed* from the small bowel, (b) *excreted* through the liver in a similar fashion to bilirubin (following conjugation), and then (c) *concentrated* by the gallbladder (maximal concentration occurs 14 to 16 hours after ingestion of Telepaque, 6 to 8 hours with Oragrafin). An unexplained 20 to 25 per cent of subsequently normal patients will show poor visualization or nonvisualization of the gallbladder following a single dose of Telepaque and will require a *repeat* dose of six tablets (3 grams) (the unfortunately misnamed "double dose" cholecystogram). It is important not to give a

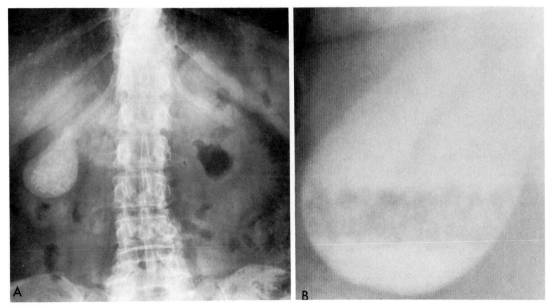

Figure 13–4. *A*, On a supine film, following administration of oral cholecystographic contrast, the opacified gallbladder in the right upper quadrant is seen to have multiple tiny filling defects within it representing nonopaque calculi. Although these defects are obvious, smaller calculi may not be visible at all in the supine position and that is why erect films are obtained. *B*, An erect film shows layering of myriad tiny stones, the stones finding their own level in the bile and contrast medium, depending on their specific gravity.

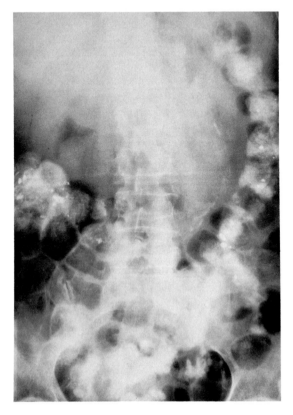

Figure 13–5. There is both unabsorbed (dense white and clumpy) contrast and absorbed and re-excreted (hazy and amorphous) contrast material in the colon. Incidentally, notice the large aortic aneurysm (the curvilinear calcifications delineating both walls of the aorta).

double dose (i.e., 12 tablets) at one time because this much contrast medium is uricosuric and nephrotoxic; acute tubular necrosis has been produced in a few patients who had unsuspected renal impairment.

Films of the right upper quadrant are taken with the patient both horizontal and erect (Fig. 13–4), with compression for adequate penetration. If overlying gas or feces is a problem, a decubitus film may be used; occasionally even a washout enema may be necessary.

If the gallbladder is not seen in the right upper quadrant, a full KUB is necessary to exclude a very low or even ectopic gallbladder. If the gallbladder is still not seen, it may be

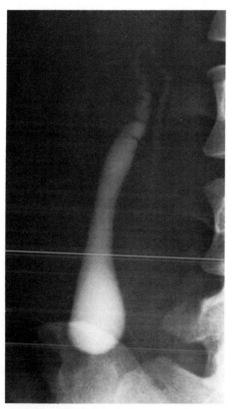

Figure 13–6. *Normal gallbladder following fatty meal.* There is good opacification of the gallbladder and the spiral valves of Heister are well demonstrated within the cystic duct. As this is a post–fatty meal film, there is some contrast medium seen within the common bile duct. With some of the newer oral cholecystographic agents, e.g., Solubiloptin and Biloptin, visualization of the common bile duct is quite usual even without a fatty meal.

TABLE 13–2. INDICATIONS FOR FATTY MEAL

1. A large, floppy gallbladder (dyskinesia?)
2. Suspected adenomyomatosis (this may be obvious only after contraction of the gallbladder—a fuzzy appearance may suggest it before the fatty meal is given)
3. Inability to remove overlying gas by positioning—contraction of the gallbladder may displace it away from the offending gas
4. Overopacification of the gallbladder—following contraction of the gallbladder and evacuation of some of the contrast medium, adequate compression and penetration may be obtained

Note: Do not give patients with known gallstones a fatty meal or you may precipitate biliary colic!

because it is indeed diseased or because the contrast agent was never properly absorbed and excreted. If absorbed and reexcreted contrast medium can be identified in the bowel (Fig. 13–5), the conclusion can be made that the gallbladder is diseased. Tomograms of the right upper quadrant may be helpful in searching for other clues of gallbladder disease. These include the faint calcifications of stones impacted in the gallbladder neck or nonvisualization of the gallbladder despite opacification of the common bile duct.

With *oral* contrast media usually only the gallbladder can be examined because the contrast is not excreted by the liver in a high enough concentration to be visible; not even the gallbladder will be visible until there is further concentration by the gallbladder itself.

Cholecystokinin (CCK) Cholangiogram

A fatty meal can be given to assess gallbladder contraction (Fig. 13–6) and may be useful under certain other circumstances (Table 13–2). A variant of the fatty meal is the cholecystokinin (CCK) cholangiogram. Injection of this hormone causes gallbladder contraction, as does the ingestion of a fatty meal, but its effect is more predictable. It is especially useful in a patient who is scheduled for both an OCG and an upper GI series the same day. CCK has been advocated as a test for biliary dyskinesia, but it should be stressed

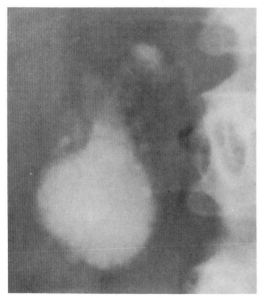

Figure 13–7. *Adenomyomatosis.* There are multiple tiny, rounded collections of contrast medium extending from and paralleling the wall of the gallbladder; this is due to contrast medium within dilated Rokitansky-Aschoff sinuses.

that many authorities are skeptical of the existence of such an entity, and the provocative CCK test has fallen into some disfavor. Please note that CCK is contraindicated in acute pancreatitis, as it also stimulates pancreatic secretion.

Intravenous Cholangiogram (IVC)

The *intravenous cholangiogram* (IVC) may be useful if duct pathology is suspected, in the postcholecystectomy patient, if the patient has vomited oral contrast, or in the "failed OCG." Contrast medium (Cholografin) is given intravenously at a rate adequate to ensure maximum transport within the liver but not so rapidly that reactions such as nausea or vomiting occur. Two common methods are injection over 10 minutes or infusion over 30 minutes, with most now favoring a slow infusion. The contrast medium is excreted by the liver in a high enough concentration to visualize the common bile duct and the main intrahepatic ducts (Fig. 13–8), although tomography will usually be necessary.

Tomograms are taken as required, usually

after at least 30 minutes. Normally the common bile duct is seen first and as time proceeds, the intrahepatic radicles fill. If this time sequence is reversed, and the intrahepatic radicles are seen first, there is slow bile flow, which is an early clue to obstruction; by extending the study until adequate opacification is obtained complete and partial obstruction can be differentiated.

Passive gallbladder opacification occurs if the cystic duct is patent, eventually allowing assessment of the gallbladder (films as for OCG). Although the ducts are seen early (30 to 60 min), the gallbladder may take up to 6 or even 24 hours to be adequately opacified (the patient remains on fat-free diet until all gallbladder films are taken). In acute cholecystitis, the gallbladder will not fill, as the underlying pathology is cystic duct obstruction. Since in some normal patients the gallbladder may take up to 24 hours to fill, diagnosis may be de-

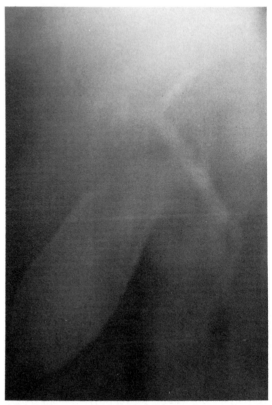

Figure 13–8. *Normal intravenous cholangiogram.* There is excellent visualization of a normal common bile duct. Since the cystic duct is patent, the gallbladder has filled passively.

layed in this condition for many hours. For this reason, faster diagnostic modalities are preferred in suspected cases of acute cholecystitis; these will be described later.

Normal measurements for the common bile duct have been established; <8 mm or >14 mm is definitely abnormal; between 8 and 14 mm is a "gray zone," where other criteria have to be applied if the clinical question is whether or not there is partial obstruction.

Even with a normal serum bilirubin level, there is an unexplained failure of duct visualization in approximately 6 per cent of patients; the success rate decreases dramatically as the bilirubin concentration increases, e.g., with a bilirubin of 4 mg/dl, adequate opacification can be expected in only 10 per cent of patients. At this bilirubin level, other diagnostic tools should be chosen.

The side effects of the IVC in general are mild and related to the speed of the injection and the dose of contrast medium. Serious contrast reactions, however, may occur; the mortality rate is 1 in 5000 patients, approximately eight times the death rate following intravenous urographic contrast media.

If the patient is *jaundiced,* none of the previously mentioned techniques will be adequate; some way then has to be found to evaluate the size of the biliary tree and to define the anatomy related to it. The following discussion lists some of the ways available.

Percutaneous Cholangiography (PCC)

This is an interventional technique that gained a poor reputation in its early years. It was then performed with a wide-bore (16 gauge) needle, and many complications resulted, the most serious of which were severe hemorrhage and bile peritonitis. Many patients went directly from the x-ray table to the operating room for emergency surgery following the examination; operating room time had to be available.

Since the introduction of the Chiba needle (23 gauge), this test is no longer as dangerous. The complication rate has decreased dramatically to approximately 1 per cent. While

being monitored fluoroscopically and with respiration suspended, the needle is inserted into the liver via a lateral axillary approach (by using the lateral approach the ribs can serve as a splint, and the method is far safer than the old anterior approach). Contrast medium is injected while slowly withdrawing the needle (it is too fine to aspirate bile through). Since this is a "blind" technique, arteries, veins, and even lymph channels may be entered. When ducts are seen, contrast medium is injected to identify the site and cause of the obstruction (Fig. 13–9). A tilting table is a vital part of this study to enable the level of the obstruction to be found without overdistending the ducts; the incidence of septicemia following the PCC appears to be related to overdistention of an already dilated and infected system.

Contraindications to this study are contrast allergy, bleeding diathesis (check the platelet count and PTT beforehand; correct if necessary), ascites, and severe sepsis. The success rate of duct entry is almost 100 per cent if ducts are dilated and 60 to 70 per cent with ducts of normal size. Failure to enter a duct (after at least six to eight good passes) is presumptive evidence that the ducts are not obstructed.

This diagnostic tool is especially useful in suspected bile duct disease in those patients in whom no mass is found in the head of the pancreas. Noting the way the duct terminates is helpful in differentiating among obstructing calculus, carcinoma, and chronic pancreatitis.

Endoscopic Retrograde Cholangiopancreatography (ERCP)

Another direct way to define the biliary tree is by ERCP (Fig. 13–10). The advantage of this over PCC is that the pancreatic duct may be injected at the same time; biopsies or brushings may also be taken. Depending on the skill of the examiner, cannulation is successful 70 to 80 per cent of the time for pancreatic duct, slightly less for the common bile duct. Contraindications are acute pancreatitis, active hepatitis, tuberculosis, bleeding diath-

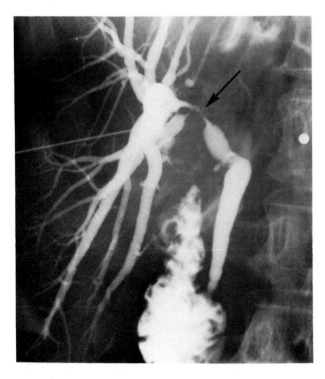

Figure 13–9. *Cholangiocarcinoma* (Klatskin tumor). On this percutaneous cholangiogram a stricture (arrow) at the bifurcation of the right and left intrahepatic ducts is seen, with nonfilling of the left intrahepatic system. The stricture also involves another intrahepatic radicle, with dilatation behind indicating partial obstruction. Because this stricture involves multiple ducts rather than a single one, this suggests malignant involvement; do not let its benign appearance fool you.

esis, and contrast allergy. Care must be taken not to overdistend the ducts by overinjection because then the complication rate (chemical pancreatitis) will rise dramatically. With this technique, obstruction of the biliary tree is tackled from below. Examination of the pancreatic duct may show evidence of chronic pancreatitis, or the duct may be obstructed by a carcinoma or calculus.

Infusion Tomography of the Gallbladder

This technique, based on the total body opacification effect, gained early popularity as a fast, easy way to diagnose acute cholecystitis; it has since become unfashionable. It was believed that a thick (greater than 1 to 2 mm) rim of contrast medium in the right upper quadrant indicated acute inflammation of the gallbladder (the rim being the inflamed wall). Subsequent studies have questioned the specificity of this finding. It must be stressed that with this technique only the thickness of the gallbladder wall can be measured; because Renografin, rather than biliary contrast medium is being used, the biliary tree is not opacified, and nonopaque gallstones will not be seen. Of course, nowadays gallbladder wall thickness can also be evaluated with ultrasound.

Isotope Scanning

One of the earliest isotopes, ^{131}I rose bengal, was used to differentiate between obstructive and nonobstructive jaundice. As newer radiopharmaceuticals have become available, this isotope has been superseded. The latest in a long line of biliary agents are the IDA (most commonly used agent, HIDA) and PYG derivatives, which even at high bilirubin levels will permit rapid evaluation of the patency of the biliary tree. A normal scan will show isotope in the gallbladder and duodenum less than 1 hour following IV injection (Fig. 13–11); slower transit will be seen in jaundiced patients. If the common bile duct is patent and contrast agent is seen in the duodenum but the gallbladder does not fill, acute cholecystitis may be assumed. At present, HIDA scanning is thought to be the most rapid and accurate way to diagnose acute cholecystitis (98 per cent accurate). It can also be extremely helpful in biliary obstruction or bile leaks. Of course, owing to the poor resolution of the gamma camera, calculi will not be seen, and although the *level* of an obstruction will be defined, what is causing that obstruction will have to be determined by other means (ultrasound, CT, PCC, or ERCP).

Intraoperative Cholangiography

This is performed by injecting contrast medium through the cystic duct remnant. Any calculi in the common bile duct or the intrahepatic radicles will be seen, and the stones can be extracted then and there. Some surgeons do not do this routinely, but it is

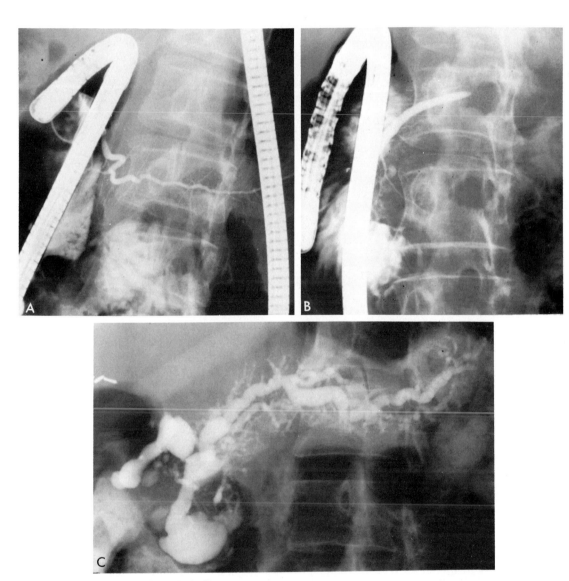

Figure 13–10. *A range of ERCP findings.*

A, The normal pancreatic duct tapers as it extends outward toward the hilus of the spleen. The side branches are fine and regular.

B, There is abrupt termination of the main pancreatic duct in a "rat-tail" appearance; this is characteristic of *carcinoma.*

C, Chronic pancreatitis. Both the main and side branches are ectatic; this is characteristic of chronic pancreatitis. The larger collections represent pseudocysts.

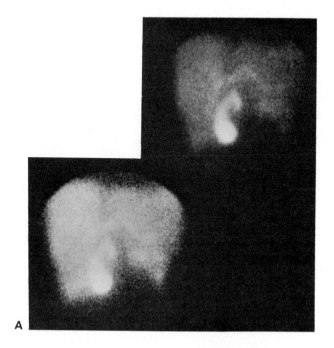

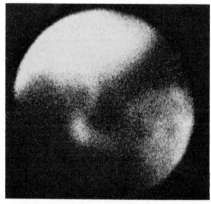

Figure 13–11. *HIDA Scans. A,* A normal HIDA scan at 30 minutes, with isotope in the gallbladder as well as in the bowel. *B,* Compare this abnormal scan with the normal; at 1½ hours, there is still no isotope in the gallbladder although the biliary tree and duodenum are seen. This implies cystic duct obstruction and indicates acute cholecystitis.

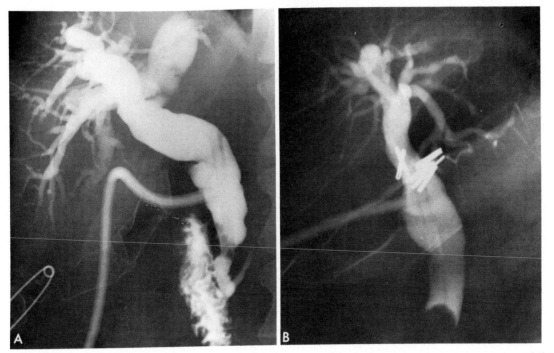

Figure 13–12. *A, Retained calculi.* A T-tube cholangiogram demonstrates dilatation of the common bile duct (due to partial obstruction); note the small retained calculi in the distal duct.

B, The "pseudocalculus sign." No stone is present, but spasm of the sphincter of Oddi simulates the meniscus sign. Glucagon may be helpful in distinguishing between pseudo-obstruction due to spasm and a real calculus.

certainly easier to deal with these calculi at surgery than later (when they are known as *retained calculi*) (Fig. 13–12).

One week postcholecystectomy, a *T-tube cholangiogram* is done for two main reasons: (1) to look for any retained calculi; and (2) to make sure, before removing the T-tube, that there is no obstruction to flow of bile into the duodenum (especially important if bougies were passed at surgery and the ampulla traumatized).

It is important to inject contrast medium slowly, with careful fluoroscopy; if the injection pressure is too high, the sphincter will go into spasm, the patient will experience pain, and a false-positive diagnosis of obstruction may be made (Fig. 13–12). As with percutaneous cholangiography, overdistention of the biliary tree should be avoided.

The intrahepatic ducts should be filled first. It may be necessary to put the patient in the Trendelenburg position and with the left side to the table to fill the left system. Unless all the intrahepatic radicles are filled, the study is incomplete because retained intrahepatic calculi cannot be excluded. The common bile duct is then studied.

If retained calculi are found, there are a number of approaches possible. An attempt can be made to dissolve the calculi by infusing chenodeoxycholic acid or heparin into the T-tube, and this may be successful with cholesterol stones, although it is a prolonged process. Another approach is to do a papillotomy (cutting the papilla via ERCP), hoping the stones will fall through into the duodenum. If they do not, one can pass a basket up through the now open papilla and attempt to grab them. An alternative procedure, especially if the stones are in the hepatic ducts, is basket extraction with a steerable catheter through the matured T-tube tract. Both these methods are attractive alternatives to reoperation in cases of retained stones.

TABLE 13–3. BILIARY/PANCREATIC DECISION TREE

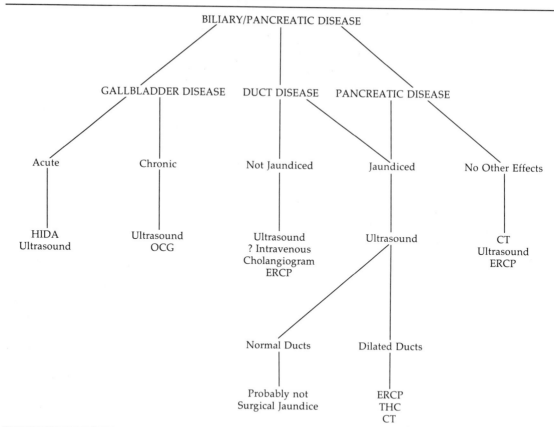

RECOMMENDATIONS FOR SOME CLINICAL SITUATIONS (Table 13–3)

1. *Chronic pain in the right upper quadrant* (thought to be due to gallstones). Many would now recommend ultrasound as the initial screening procedure in these cases and would suggest that it replace the oral cholecystogram. Others would perform ultrasound if a single dose of oral contrast medium did not result in adequate visualization. (It has been estimated that this approach would save $12 million per year in the United States in contrast medium costs alone.)

2. *Acute right upper quadrant pain and fever.* This symptom complex is most likely the result of *acute cholecystitis*. In past years, nonvisualization of the gallbladder following two consecutive doses of oral contrast medium (2 days to complete) or failure to visualize the gallbladder following a successful intravenous cholangiogram (up to 24 hours to complete) would have been two ways to make this diagnosis. Today more rapid and accurate techniques are available. Opinion is divided between ultrasound and HIDA scanning as the preferred initial diagnostic test, with many giving the edge to HIDA.

3. *The jaundiced patient.* In this patient, it is necessary to determine whether or not the biliary tree is dilated (Fig. 13–13). The procedure of choice is ultrasound, since it is both noninvasive and highly accurate. This may be the only test necessary if the cause for any duct dilatation is also found, e.g., enlargement of the head of the pancreas. Failure to demonstrate a cause for dilatation or equivocal results on ultrasound necessitates undertaking other investigations. If ultrasound is unsuccessful, CT may be done. CT can diagnose dilated ducts and may locate the cause, such as a pancreatic mass. If ultrasound shows dilated ducts but no cause for them, the biliary tree may be defined by contrast medium injection,

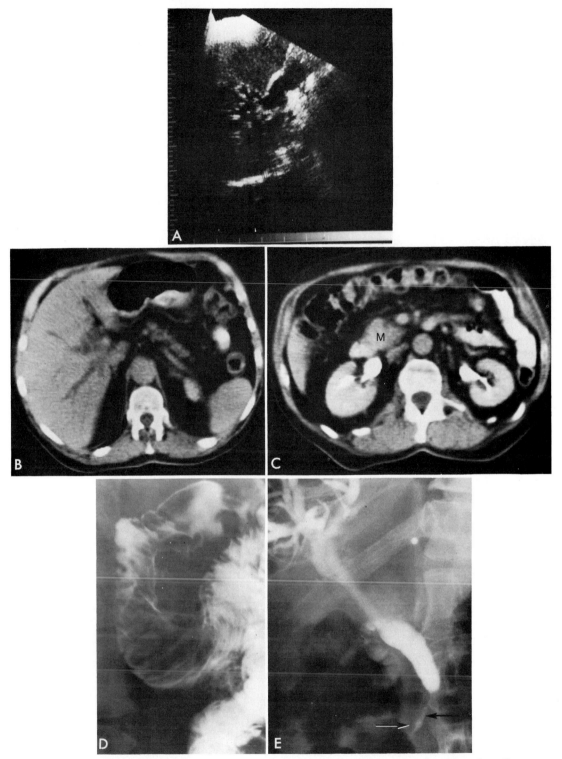

Figure 13–13. *The jaundiced patient.* A 43 year old man with the acute onset of painless jaundice.

A–C, Ultrasound *(A)* shows dilated intra- and extrahepatic ducts, these findings being confirmed by CT *(B)*. A lower cut *(C)* shows the mass *(M)* in the pancreatic head responsible for the obstruction.

D, An upper GI series shows the "reverse 3" sign with invasion, straightening, and rigidity of the inner aspect of the C-sweep; these findings indicate carcinoma.

E, Percutaneous cholangiogram shows irregular narrowing of the extreme distal common bile duct (arrows); remember that the distal common bile duct runs through the pancreas before it enters the duodenum. The irregularity here favors the diagnosis of carcinoma rather than involvement by pancreatitis.

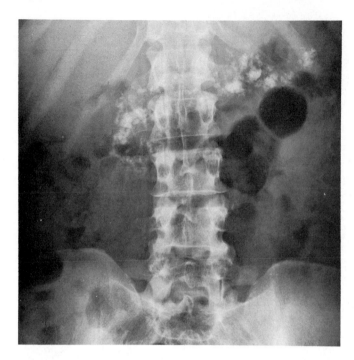

Figure 13–14. *Calcific pancreatitis.* There are multiple calcifications in the shape of the pancreas owing to alcoholic pancreatitis.

either PCC or ERCP; which test is chosen depends on the clinical setting and local expertise with these more invasive procedures.

In general, in the jaundiced patient the intravenous cholangiogram will not be successful and should not even be attempted: direct visualization is indicated.

THE PANCREAS

The pancreas is an extremely inaccessible organ to physical examination. Pancreatic disease may cause jaundice early ("painless jaundice") if it involves the head of the pancreas, but, it unfortunately, may be extremely silent

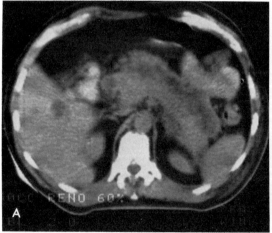
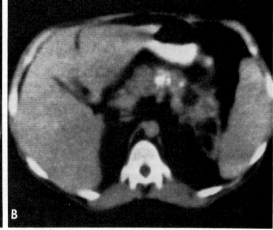

Figure 13–15. *Pancreatitis. A,* Computed tomography through the pancreas shows diffuse enlargement of the pancreas consistent with phlegmonous pancreatitis. The contrast-containing duodenal C-sweep is displaced laterally by the enlargement. The filling defect within the liver is not a metastasis but represents the gallbladder.

B, Computed tomography of acute-on-chronic pancreatitis shows calcification and areas of lower attenuation, which are small pseudocysts.

and present too late to be treatable if the body or tail is diseased. In the past, barium studies played an important role in the search for pancreatic disease (Fig. 13–16); the signs sought were duodenal abnormalities (enlarge-ment, inflammation, or invasion) or displace-ment of the stomach or ligament of Treitz. Two other views are useful in diagnosing pancreatic disease. The cross-table lateral view may show anterior displacement of the

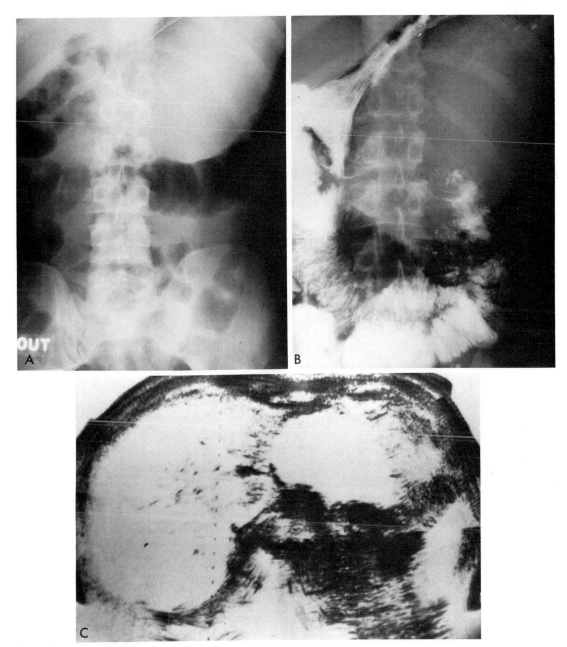

Figure 13–16. *Pancreatic pseudocyst.*
  A, Plain film shows wide separation of the stomach and transverse colon due to a large pseudocyst extending into the gastrocolic ligament.
  B, With barium, the displacement and extrinsic mass effect are even more obvious.
  C, Ultrasonic scan shows the large central anechoic area of the pseudocyst.

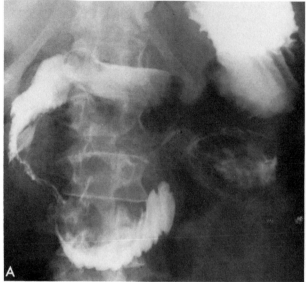

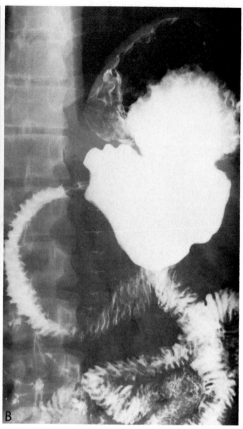

Figure 13–17. *Carcinoma of the pancreas. A,* In addition to enlargement of the C-sweep by mass effect, with the double contour due to a mass in the pancreatic head seen best on the horizontal limb of the duodenum, there is also complete destruction of the mucosa in the descending limb. *B,* Compare this appearance with that in another patient. The C-sweep is also enlarged; here, however, the folds are intact but thick, owing to inflammation. This latter patient had *acute pancreatitis.*

stomach. The "stooping lateral" view will demonstrate that a normal stomach can flop forward when the patient bends over; a fixed stomach will not do this.

Oral contrast studies have been superseded by the advent of ultrasound and CT (Figs. 13–15, 13–16). The pancreas and retroperitoneum may be successfully studied by either technique, although ultrasound is limited by overlying intestinal gas and obesity. CT is able to visualize the pancreas in most patients, especially the obese, and is not hindered by intestinal gas. Barium within the gut, however, is a problem with both techniques. Because of this, ultrasound or CT should be performed before any contrast study.

Both methods can tell whether there is a localized mass or diffuse enlargement. Diffuse enlargement suggests pancreatitis (Fig. 13–15), but differentiation between *localized* pancreatitis and a mass due to carcinoma is frequently impossible. ERCP or biopsy is indicated when faced with this problem.

Complications of pancreatitis (pseudocyst, abscess) will be clearly revealed by either CT or ultrasound.

If no mass is seen with cross-sectional imaging techniques, the pancreatic duct may be studied by ERCP and, at the same time, brushing and biopsy can be performed. The ectasia of chronic pancreatitis, or blockage of the duct ("rat-tailing") due to carcinoma, may be defined.

Radionuclide examination of the pancreas has proved disappointing and has been superseded by CT and ultrasound.

References

General

Baker DH, Gorson RO, Lalli A, Moseley RD Jr: Problem areas in the biliary tract. Curr Probl Radiol 5:44, 1975.
Gastrointestinal Radiology (Special Issue) 3:243–353, 1978.

Leopold GR: Ultrasonography of jaundice. Radiol Clin North Am 17:127–136, 1979.

Levitt RG, Geisse GG, Sagel SS, Stanley RJ, Evens RG, Koehler RE, Josr RG: Complementary use of ultrasound and computed tomography in studies of the pancreas and kidney. Radiology 126:149–152, 1978.

Sample WF, Sarti DA, Goldstein LI, Weiner M, Kadell BM: Gray-scale ultrasonography of the jaundiced patient. Radiology 128:719–725, 1978.

Seltzer SE, Jones B: Imaging the hepatobiliary system in acute disease. Am J Roentgenol 135:407–416, 1980.

Gallbladder

Anderson JC, Harned RK: Gray scale ultrasonography of the gallbladder: an evaluation of accuracy and report of additional ultrasound signs. Am J Roentgenol 129:973–978, 1977.

Anderson JF, Madsen PER: The value of plain radiographs prior to oral cholecystography. Radiology 133:309–310, 1979.

Berk RN, Clemett AR: Radiology of the Gallbladder and Bile Ducts. Philadelphia, WB Saunders Co, 1977.

The gallbladder and biliary tract. I. Methodology. Semin Roentgenol 11:147–230, 1976.

The gallbladder and biliary tract. II. Diseases. Semin Roentgenol 11:235–287, 1976.

Harley WD, Kirkpatrick RH, Ferrucci JT: Gas in bile ducts (pneumobilia) in emphysematous cholecystitis. Am J Roentgenol 131:661–663, 1978.

Jutras JA, Lévesque HP: Adenomyoma and adenomyomatosis of the gallbladder: radiologic and pathologic correlations. Radiol Clin North Am 4:483–500, 1966.

Jutras JA, Longtin, JM, Lévesque HP: Hyperplastic cholecystoses. Hickey Lecture 1960. Am J Roentgenol 83:795–827, 1960.

Love L, Kucharski P, Pickelman J: Radiology of cholecystectomy complications. Gastrointest Radiol 4:33–40, 1979.

McIntosh DMF, Penney H: Gray-scale ultrasonography as a screening procedure in the detection of gallbladder disease. Radiology 136:725–727, 1980.

Manzione JV, Braver JM: Imaging the Gallbladder 1981. Postgrad Radiol (in press).

Ochsner F: Adenomyoma of the gallbladder. Am J Roentgenol 88:778–782, 1962.

Schein CJ: Acute Cholecystitis. New York, Harper & Row, 1972.

Wise RE: Intravenous Cholangiography. Springfield, Ill, Charles C Thomas, 1962.

Liver

Black EB, Ferrucci JT Jr: New cholangiographic sign of common bile duct obstruction: initial opacification of intrahepatic ducts. Am J Roentgenol 130:61–65, 1978.

Buonocore E: Transhepatic percutaneous cholangiography. Radiol Clin North Am 14:527–542, 1975.

Burhenne HJ: Nonoperative extraction of stones from the bile ducts. Semin Roentgenol 11:213–217, 1976.

Burhenne HJ: Garland lecture: percutaneous extraction of retained biliary tract stones: 661 patients. Am J Roentgenol 134:888–898, 1980.

Ferrucci JT Jr, Wittenberg J, Sarno RA, Dreyfuss JR: Fine needle transhepatic cholangiography: a new approach to obstructive jaundice. Am J Roentgenol 127:403–407, 1976.

Kattan KR: Symposium on noninvasive radiology of the liver. Radiol Clin North Am 18:179–338, 1980.

The liver. Semin Roentgenol 10:169–244, 1975.

Menuck L, Amberg J: The bile ducts. Radiol Clin North Am 14:499, 1976.

Molnar W, Stockum AE: Transhepatic dilatation of choledochoenterostomy strictures. Radiology 129:59–64, 1978.

New procedure for removing gallstones without surgery. Resident and Staff Physician 24:116–117, 1978.

Pereiras R, Schiff E, Barkin J, Hutson D: The role of interventional radiology in diseases of the hepatobiliary system and the pancreas. Radiol Clin North Am 17:555–606, 1979.

Petasnick JP, Ram P, Turner DA, Fordham EW: The relationship of computed tomography, gray-scale ultrasonography and radionuclide imaging in the evaluation of hepatic masses. Semin Nucl Med 9:8–21, 1979.

Scholz FJ, Johnston DO, Wise RE: Intravenous cholangiography: optimum dosage and methodology. Radiology 114:513–518, 1975.

Pancreas

Balthazar EJ: Radiological signs of acute pancreatitis. CRC Crit Rev Clin Radiol Nucl Med 7:199, 1975.

Davis S, Parbhoo SP, Gibson MJ: The plain abdominal radiograph in acute pancreatitis. Clin Radiol 31:87–93, 1980.

Ferrucci JT Jr: Radiology of the pancreas, 1976. Sonography and ductography. Radiol Clin North Am 14:543–562, 1976.

Foley WD, Stewart ET, Lawson TL, Greenan J, Loguidice J, Mahler L, Unger GF: Computed tomography, ultrasonography and endoscopic retrograde cholangiopancreatography in the diagnosis of pancreatic disease: a comparative study. Gastrointest Radiol 5:29–36, 1980.

Haaga JR, Alfidi RJ, Zelch MG, Meany TF, Boller M, Gonzales L, Jelden GL: Computed tomography of the pancreas. Radiology 120:589–596, 1976.

Komaki S, Clark JM: Pancreatic pseudocyst: a review of 17 cases with emphasis on radiologic findings. Am J Roentgenol 122:385, 1974.

Kressel HY, Margulis AR, Gooding GW, Filly RA, Moss AA, Korobkin M: CT scanning and ultrasound in the evaluation of pancreatic pseudocysts: a preliminary comparison. Radiology 126:153–157, 1978.

Lee JKT, Stanley RJ, Melson GL, Sagel SS: Pancreatic imaging by ultrasound and computed tomography: a general review. Radiol Clin North Am 17:105–118, 1979.

Moreno G, Rivera HH: Evaluation of the gastrocolic space in 100 cases of acute pancreatitis. Radiology 118:535–538, 1976.

Nix GAJJ: Early carcinoma of the ampulla and papilla of vater. Clin Radiol 31:95–100, 1980.

Paul RE Jr: Endoscopic retrograde cholangiography. Semin Roentgenol 11:223–226, 1976.

Rohrmann CA, Silvis SE, Vennes JA: Evaluation of the endoscopic pancreatogram. Radiology 113:297–304, 1974.

Rohrmann CA Jr, Silvis SE, Vennes JA: The significance of pancreatic ductal obstruction in differential diagnosis of the abnormal endoscopic retrograde pancreatogram. Radiology 131:311–314, 1976.

Scholz FJ, Matfield PM, Larsen CR, Wise RE: Carcinoma of the pancreas. Curr Probl Radiol 7:4–41, 1977.

Siegel JH: ERCP update: diagnostic and therapeutic applications. Gastrointest Radiol 3:311–318, 1978.

Sivak MV Jr, Sullivan BH Jr: Endoscopic retrograde pancreatography. Digest Dis 21:263–269, 1976.

Stone L, Eaton SB Jr, Ferrucci JT Jr.: Inflammatory disease of the pancreas. Curr Probl Radiol 5:3–43, 1975.

Thoeni RF, Gedgaudas RK: Ectopic pancreas: usual and unusual features. Gastrointest Radiol 5:37–42, 1980.

Varley PF, Rohrmann CA Jr, Silvis SE, Vennes JA: The normal endoscopic pancreatogram. Radiology 118:295–300, 1976.

Viamonte M Jr: Morphologic-radiographic correlations of the pancreas. Radiol Clin North Am 17:119–126, 1979.

INDEX

Numbers in *italics* denote illustrations; (t) refers to tabular material.